Danilo Peron Meireles
Alessandra C. Goulart

The Prognostic Value of Carotid Intima-Media Thickness

Danilo Peron Meireles
Alessandra C. Goulart

The Prognostic Value of Carotid Intima-Media Thickness

Study of short- and long-term mortality in the ERICO acute coronary insufficiency registry strategy

ScienciaScripts

Imprint

Any brand names and product names mentioned in this book are subject to trademark, brand or patent protection and are trademarks or registered trademarks of their respective holders. The use of brand names, product names, common names, trade names, product descriptions etc. even without a particular marking in this work is in no way to be construed to mean that such names may be regarded as unrestricted in respect of trademark and brand protection legislation and could thus be used by anyone.

Cover image: www.ingimage.com

This book is a translation from the original published under ISBN 978-613-9-61309-0.

Publisher:
Sciencia Scripts
is a trademark of
Dodo Books Indian Ocean Ltd. and OmniScriptum S.R.L publishing group

120 High Road, East Finchley, London, N2 9ED, United Kingdom
Str. Armeneasca 28/1, office 1, Chisinau MD-2012, Republic of Moldova, Europe
Printed at: see last page
ISBN: 978-620-7-63452-1

Table of contents:

DEDICATION

To my dear parents, Geraldo and Margarida, who, despite the lack of formal education in their lives, established education and knowledge as priorities in the creation and consolidation of their family.

To my brother, Geraldo, for his companionship.

To my wife, Diane, who gave up some of her dreams to make this work a reality, and especially to my son, Lorenzo, who has always been my greatest source of inspiration.

ACKNOWLEDGMENTS

First of all to God for guiding me and giving me strength in the most difficult times.

To my advisor **Prof®. Dr.ª . Alessandra Carvalho Goulart**, for accepting me as her student, for her patience and teachings during this period, as well as for the time she gave me and for emphasizing that without her participation, all this work would not have been completed.

To professors and friends **Nelson Bergman Sanchez Muñoz** and **Amaury de Castro Júnior** who, together with **Prof® Dr® Ilka Regina Souza de Oliveira,** gave me the opportunity to enter the field of research and all their teachings, especially about my introduction to the ultrasound method, as well as the professional and personal teachings that I will carry with me throughout my life.

To the radiologists who helped me throughout my learning process, **Dr. Brenda Margatho Ramos Martines, Dr.⁰ Joao Augusto Martines** and **Dr. Márcia Etsuko Kuroishi,** for the knowledge they passed on to me during long and fun days of analyzing ultrasound images.

To Professors Drs. **Paulo Andrade Lotufo** and **Isabela Judith Martins Benseñor** who allowed me to participate in all the studies carried out at the Clinical and Epidemiological Research Center of the University Hospital of USP, as well as their trust in my work specifically at the Ultrasound Reading Center of the ELSA-Brazil Project.

To **Prof. Dr. Itamar de Souza Santos** for accompanying and developing the studies on intima-media thickness, as well as the biostatistics classes together with **Prof. Dr. Itamar de Souza Santos. Prof® Drª Alessandra Carvalho Goulart**.

The examining board for my qualification, Professors **Airlane Alencar, Itamar Santos** and **Paulo Lotufo,** for their contributions, suggestions and improvements to this dissertation.

To all my friends at the Clinical and Epidemiological Research Center of the University Hospital of the University of Sao Paulo and the Nove de Julho University, who contributed during my journey in this endeavor.

To the 1085 participants of the ERICO Project, whose contribution has enabled this work to be carried out and has allowed the frontiers of clinical research in Brazil to be expanded.

And to all the family and friends who have contributed in some way to this work.

SUMMARY

Meireles DP. *Prognostic value of carotid artery intima-media thickness in short- and long-term mortality in the acute coronary syndrome registry strategy (ERICO)* [Dissertation]. Sao Paulo: School of Medicine, University of Sao Paulo; 2017.

INTRODUCTION: Atherosclerosis in the carotid arteries can determine a poor prognosis in individuals after the occurrence of acute coronary syndrome (ACS). Therefore, we sought to assess mortality associated with carotid intima-media thickness (CIMT) in participants in the Acute Coronary Syndrome Registry Strategy (ACSR) study. **METHODS:** CIMT was assessed by B-mode ultrasound to evaluate the risk of mortality at 180 days, 1, 2 and 3 years. We performed Kaplan-Meier survival curves and Cox logistic regression models to assess all-cause mortality, cardiovascular disease (CVD) and coronary artery disease (CAD) by tertiles of EMIC in crude, age- and sex-adjusted and multivariate-adjusted models. **RESULTS:** Among 644 individuals with ACS (mean age 61 years), we observed a median CIMT of 0.74 mm (0.40-1.90). In addition to aging, lower education, hypertension, diabetes and dyslipidemia were associated with higher CIMT values (3° tertile: 0.81-1.90 mm). During 3 years of follow-up, we observed 65 deaths (10.1%), crude case fatality rates were progressively higher in the EMIC tertiles in all periods, with the highest rates observed in participants with the highest EMIC (3 tertile) (180 days: 6.6% *vs.* 1 year: 9.0% *vs.* 2 years: 12.3% *vs.* 3 years: 16.0%, P <0.05). In the crude analyses, lower survival rates (all-cause, CVD and CAD, *p log-rank* values <0.005) and higher hazard ratios for death for all-cause and CVD (from 1 to 3 years) and for CAD (2 and 3 years) were observed. However, we did not maintain significant results after adjusting for age. **CONCLUSION**: EMIC was mainly influenced by aging. EMIC was not a good predictor of all-cause mortality, CVD or CAD in the ERICO study.

Keywords: carotid intima-media thickness; coronary artery disease; cardiovascular diseases; prognosis; survival.

Chapter 1

1. INTRODUCTION

1.1 Identifying the problem

The group of cardiovascular diseases (CVD) is responsible for the largest cause of mortality in the world. In particular, ischemic heart disease is still the leading cause of mortality for both sexes, showing an increase of 19%, from 7.9 million deaths in 2006 to 9.4 million deaths in 2016 (GBD, 2016). It is estimated that by 2030 there will be more than double the number of deaths from CVD and the most affected countries will continue to be developing countries, including Brazil (WHO, 2011; Yusuf et al, 2014; Vos et al, 2015; WHO, 2016).

According to recent data from the Ministry of Health, 31% of all deaths that occurred in 2011 were due to CVD, and of these deaths, 31.1% were due to coronary artery disease (CAD) (Ribeiro et al, 2016). National statistics show that age-adjusted mortality rates for CVD decreased by 24% between 2000 and 2011, with a slower decline in mortality rates for men compared to women (Ribeiro et al, 2016; Lotufo et al, 2013).

Early identification of cardiovascular risk factors, including carotid atherosclerosis, is extremely important, as it will allow treatments to be targeted and applied before a recurrent event or death occurs in a population at increased cardiovascular risk, such as individuals with acute coronary syndrome (ACS).

The underlying pathophysiology of CAD is the chronic and progressive atherosclerotic process, which corroborates systemic inflammation and affects all arterial walls, so the estimated risk of CIMT obtained from the carotid artery can predict the occurrence of CAD (Toth, 2008).

The development of intima-media thickening in the artery is directly related to ageing and the presence of cardiovascular risk factors (CVRF), beginning years before clinical events develop in a stage called subclinical atherosclerosis (Koskinen et al, 2009; Toth, 2008). Atherosclerotic plaques are slowly progressive, beginning with the transport of low-density lipoproteins through the endothelium into the subendothelial space. Endothelial dysfunction is characterized by an increase in the permeability of the endothelium to lipoproteins and can initiate the process of atherosclerotic plaque formation. Oxidation of LDL-cholesterol is the next step in plaque formation, triggering a local inflammatory reaction. The degree of fibroblast proliferation and the migration of smooth muscle cells from the medial layer to the subendothelial space, which is part of the atherosclerotic process, can be inferred by the carotid artery intima-media thickness (CIMT).

CIMT, which is a measurement obtained by a non-invasive method, B-mode ultrasound, which makes it possible to visualize changes from the earliest stages of atherosclerosis (Koskinen et al, 2009; Howard et al, 1993) and can thus be a good surrogate marker of subclinical atherosclerosis (O'Leary et al, 1996). The prognostic value of CIMT for predicting CVD, including CAD and stroke in individuals with a high rate of CVRF and presumed subclinical atherosclerosis has been described in some previous studies (Bots et al, 1997; Andreas et al, 2003; Chambles et al, 1997;

Lorenz et al, 2006; Peters et al, 2012; Polak et al, 2011).

In this context, EMIC is a well-described surrogate marker in cardiovascular disease and its increase has been associated with the incidence and recurrence of coronary events. In particular, the prognostic value of CIMT in relation to non-fatal and fatal cardiovascular events was assessed in the *Framingham Offspring Study* cohort over a long term (mean follow-up of 7.2 years) and both CIMT, of the common carotid artery (CCA) and internal carotid artery (ICA), were found to be significant.

good predictors of cardiovascular outcomes (Polak et al, 2011).

Therefore, it was decided to evaluate the prognostic value of CIMT in all-cause mortality, CVD and CAD during three years of follow-up among participants who survived an acute coronary event and underwent CIMT evaluation of the Coronary Heart Failure Registry Strategy (CHIS), a prospective cohort of patients seen in the Emergency Department of the University Hospital-USP (HU-USP), in an area of low socioeconomic status in the western region of the city of Sao Paulo, Brazil (Goulart et al, 2013; Santos et al, 2015).

1.2 Pathophysiology of acute coronary syndrome

Patients with ischemic heart disease are divided into two large groups of patients: (1) those with chronic coronary artery disease who have more chronic stable angina (SA) and those with acute coronary syndrome (ACS). The latter group has three subtypes: unstable angina, acute myocardial infarction without segment elevation and acute myocardial infarction with segment elevation (Longo et al, 2012).

ACS mainly results from rupture of the vulnerable plaque or superficial erosion of the endothelium. Increasing exposure to statin treatment has reduced the lipid and inflammatory content of plaques, resulting in a progressive reduction in infarcts with complete occlusion of the vessel and even recurrence of coronary events. On the other hand, with greater longevity and increasing prevalence of obesity and diabetes, endothelial erosion has become more present, especially in presentations with transient or partial coronary occlusions, suggested by the higher incidence of non-ST-segment elevation myocardial infarctions (NSTEMI) and unstable angina (UA). Advances in understanding the role of cholesterol and inflammation have provided a new therapeutic approach to acute coronary syndromes, including improved microcirculation, reduced infarct mass and better ventricular remodeling (Fonseca and Izar, 2016).

Both lipid and inflammatory mechanisms appear to be associated with vulnerable plaque complications and endothelial erosion, and the magnitude of the inflammatory response that follows vascular occlusion is a topic of great current interest due to its role in the recovery of ischemic myocardium and recurrence of outcomes, especially during the first year after an ACS (Fonseca and Izar, 2016).

1.3 Intima-media thickening and cardiovascular disease

Arterial wall thickening is part of the atherosclerosis process. Thus, it has been theorized that CIMT measurements could help predict CVD in addition to traditional risk factors. However, recommendations on the use of CIMT for CVD risk prediction are conflicting.

In recent studies, CIMT has been introduced as a surrogate endpoint for assessing the progression of atherosclerosis (Komorovsky et al, 2005) but has yet to uncover whether there is a strong association with cardiovascular events in patients with CAD (Park et al, 2013).

For some years now, several large clinical studies, such as the Atherosclerosis Risk In Communities (ARIC) study (Chambles et al, 1997), the Cardiovascular Health Study (O'Leary et al, 1992), the Rotterdam Study (Bots et al, 1997), the Malmo Diet and Cancer Study (Rosval et al, 2005), and the Carotid Atherosclerosis Progression Study (Lorenz et al, 2010) have produced similar results. However, little or no additional prognostic value was found by adding EMIC to a traditional risk factor score, such as the *Framingham Risk Score* (FRS) (Lau et al, 2008; Yeboah et al, 2012; Simon et al, 2010).

The contradictory results on the value of carotid CME in predicting CVD risk is portrayed by the conflicting results of two meta-analyses. Lorenz et al found that the relative risks of CVD events increased by 1.15 for every 0.1 mm increase in CME (Lorenz et al, 2007), while Den Ruijter et al (2012) found no significant addition to CVD event prediction when CME was added to conventional risk prediction models.

1.4 Intima-media thickening and coronary artery disease

Several studies have shown an association between CIMT and coronary artery disease. The Kuoppio Ischemic Heart Disease study, for example, showed an 11% increase in the risk of AMI with an incremental increase of 0.1 mm in CIMT (Salonen and Salonen, 1991).

Yuk et al (2015) showed that EMIC and plaque score was an important predictor of death and major cardiovascular events, even after adjusting for other cardiovascular risk factors, especially in patients with coronary artery disease.

In Western countries, MI in the bulb of the carotid artery or in the internal carotid artery is associated with AMI and MI in the common carotid artery is associated with stroke (Johnsen and Mathiesen, 2009).

Despite this inconsistency, EMIC would be a powerful surrogate marker for assessing the severity and predicting the prognosis of coronary artery disease.

Cicorella et al. (2009) investigated the usefulness of evaluating carotid ultrasound in studies to check for EMI, unstable carotid plaques and severe stenosis to predict the presence and extent of CAD in a consecutive series of 1337 patients. They retrospectively evaluated patients' coronary angiography and carotid ultrasound. EMIC greater than 0.90 mm, unstable plaque and severe stenosis (> 70%) were considerable. They found that CME greater than 0.90 mm, unstable plaque and severe carotid stenosis were associated with CAD (*odds ratio* 2.28 [1.8-2.9] (P<0.0001), 3.6 [2.3-5.7] (P <0.001) and 4.2 [2.0-8.7] (P =0.0001), respectively.

According to these results, they confirmed the usefulness of ultrasound evaluation of the carotid artery in predicting the presence and extent of CAD.

The ARIC study ("*Atherosclerosis risk in communities*") (Chambless et al, 1997), and the "Rotterdam Study" (Bots et al, 1997), two large observational studies, used the IMCE measurement to investigate the determinants of atherosclerotic disease in the general population.

The ARIC study evaluated 7,289 men and 5,552 women aged between 45 and 64 living in four communities in the USA, followed up for four to seven years (19871993). Using B-mode US, measurements were taken in the ICA, ACC and carotid bulb (CB). The main result of this study was a *hazard ratio* (HR) of 1.13 (men) and 1.29 (women) in the incidence of acute myocardial infarction (AMI) for every 0.1 mm increase in the IMT value (Chambless et al, 1997).

Similar results were later found in the Rotterdam Study, carried out between 1990 and 1993, which included 7,983 individuals aged over 55 and followed up for approximately three years (Bots et al, 1997). The risk of AMI and stroke increased proportionally to the increase in MACE. For AMI, there was an increase of 43% for each standard deviation (SD) of the MCE, odds ratio (OR) = 1.43 (95% confidence interval - 95% CI 1.16 to 1.78); for stroke, OR = 1.41 (95% CI 1.25 to 1.82) was observed (Bots et al, 1997). In 2007, Lorenz et al. published a meta-analysis that included eight observational studies, totaling 37,197 individuals followed for almost 6 years (Lorenz et al, 2007). The aim was to assess the ability of the CIMT measurement to predict AMI or stroke. The authors found that, for every 0.1mm increase in CIMT, the future risk of AMI increased by 10% to 15%, and the risk of stroke increased by 13% to 18%, consistently demonstrating that the CIMT measurement can be used to predict stroke.

IMCE as an independent predictor of cardiovascular events (Bots et al, 1997).

1.5 Evolution of intima-media thickening

Intima-media thickening is one of the characteristics of atherosclerosis, which is a chronic, progressive, inflammatory and systemic disease that affects the arterial bed and can induce coronary and cerebral ischemia, thus characterizing it as one of the main causes of morbidity, mortality and disability in industrialized countries. Involvement of the artery begins years before clinical events develop, at a stage called subclinical atherosclerosis (SCA), and is a risk factor for adverse cardiovascular events (Toth, 2008).

The atherosclerotic process is age-related, with a long and slow asymptomatic phase. Recent data show that it begins to develop early in life, from childhood and adolescence to adulthood and manifests clinically in many patients at a relatively advanced stage (Koskinen et al, 2009) and is responsible for most major cardiovascular events. Most current prevention strategies are focused on the early identification and management of established risk factors for the disease (Wang and Beydoun, 2007).

Atherosclerosis is a disease that affects all arteries and can lead to ischemia of the heart, brain or extremities (Lusis, 2000). It is the result of complex interactions between genetic and environmental factors that induce the arterial wall to respond to stimuli through the action of the endothelium, smooth muscle cells, inflammatory cells and platelets, leading to the formation of plaques. The initial stages can occur in children and young people and are silent, evolving slowly and clinical manifestations usually appear when individuals reach middle age (Blaha et al, 2011). However, the first event caused by atherosclerosis can be fatal. Recently, the importance of subclinical atherosclerosis has been increasingly recognized, which is why many studies on this subject are being carried out, evaluating CME and already developed atherosclerotic plaques together.

The early identification of atherosclerosis has unquestionably been recognized as an inflammatory disease process. Thanks to advances in imaging techniques, the characterization and measurement of these biological processes *in vivo have* become possible using a variety of methods, from simple B-mode ultrasound (US) to sophisticated magnetic resonance imaging (Wang and Beydoun, 2000).

The measurement of atherosclerotic progression is an ideal surrogate marker and predictor of future cardiovascular events. Salonen and Salonen (1991) reported that every 0.1 millimeter increase in IMT increased the risk of CAD by 11%, and maximum IMT remained a significant predictor of acute myocardial infarction (AMI).

The "gold standard" for detecting and defining the severity, extent and rate of progression of atherosclerosis is quantitative coronary angiography. However, this technique has fundamental and important limitations, and would not be suitable for screening purposes alone, as it is a more complex, invasive and risky method, due to various factors, such as the patient's exposure to ionizing radiation, the injection of a contrast medium which can cause adverse reactions, not to mention the risk of the catheterization procedure which is linked to this technique.

More recently, carotid IMT has been measured using B-mode ultrasound, which has emerged as a more accurate, low-cost and non-invasive technique for detecting atherosclerotic progression. The technique is potentially useful as a substitute for the gold standard, which is coronary angiography, and as a second option, magnetic resonance imaging, in cardiovascular outcomes studied in clinical trials, because in addition to the characteristics already mentioned, ultrasound does not preclude any type of patient from undergoing it, as angiography excludes patients with hypersensitivity to iodinated contrast medium and magnetic resonance imaging excludes patients with metal prostheses or any other ferromagnetic metal implant. The use of ultrasound can facilitate the more agile, current, safe and economical development of effective therapies (Xu et al, 2010).

To reinforce our idea, we cite In *et al*, who compared the methods of cardiac angiotomography, Doppler ultrasound and B-mode US measurement of CME and proved that they all have an excellent correlation in the detection of atherosclerosis, the latter being the simplest and cheapest method, which is why it is currently the most widely used in research and can be applied in everyday clinical practice without exposing the patient to risk (In et al, 2012).

In addition, we can mention that despite advances in pharmaceutical interventions, the number of individuals suffering from metabolic syndrome, cardiovascular morbidity and mortality rates of future generations may continue to rise, endothelial wall disruption is multifactorial, complex and precedes clinically apparent coronary and cerebrovascular disease. Thus, evaluating the reproducibility of non-invasive techniques for assessing endothelial function should allow screening of large populations and can guide interventions designed specifically to reduce an individual's cardiovascular risk (Xu et al, 2010).

Many studies have tried to develop a relatively simple and easy way to perform non-invasive measurements of atherosclerosis and each one evaluates different atherosclerotic properties, such as calcified plaques, non-calcified plaques, measurements in the internal carotid artery, carotid bulb or common carotid artery. In this study, we investigated CIMT as a marker of subclinical carotid atherosclerosis and its prognostic value (fatal and non-fatal short- and long-term outcomes) in post-ACS patients.

1.6 Imaging methods for assessing carotid intima-media thickness

Currently, various non-invasive imaging techniques are used to identify subclinical atherosclerosis in vascular beds, such as ultrasound (USG), calcium scoring by computed tomography (CT), contrast angiotomography and magnetic resonance imaging (Shah, 2010).

Specifically in relation to USG, in 1986, Italian researchers demonstrated the interesting results obtained by an *in vitro* study *in* which 18 arteries (aortas and common carotids) were evaluated by microscopic examination and compared to B-mode USG in real time (Pignli et al, 1986). These researchers described that the characteristic image of the arterial wall on B-mode USG consisted of two parallel echogenic lines separated by a hypoechogenic space (Pignoli et al, 1986). The distance between these two lines did not differ significantly from the carotid intima-media thickness (CIMT), more popularly known by the English term: "*intimai medial thickness*" (IMT), measured by anatomopathological examination (Pignoli et al, 2986; O'Leary and Bots, 2010). In fact, B-mode USG could be useful for measuring IMT in vivo. Almost 25 years after this initial description, CIMT measurement is the most widely used non-invasive technique for assessing atherosclerosis in the scientific community, with the aim of quantifying the extent of subclinical disease and monitoring changes over time (O'Leary and Bots, 2010).

However, carotid ultrasound allows the detection of atherosclerotic plaques in addition to the CIMT measurement and both are used as markers of atherosclerosis (80). While CIMT is only a quantitative measure, atherosclerotic plaques can be assessed qualitatively (echogenicity, heterogeneity - a very subjective analysis) and quantitatively (number, area and volume) (Johnsen and Mathiesen, 2009). The ARIC study (Chambless et al, 1997) and other population-based studies have basically emphasized the measurement of EIMC (Hunt et al, 2001). In these studies, less attention was paid to quantifying and characterizing atherosclerotic plaques, but both CIMT and plaques were systematically measured in order to identify associated risk factors (Hunt et al, 2001). In this respect, Bonithon-Kopp et al. (1996) demonstrated an excellent correlation between increased IMT and the presence of plaques, and their association with cardiovascular risk factors. Duncan et al. (1997) evaluated participants in the ARIC study and described that classic risk factors such as total cholesterol, LDL-cholesterol, smoking and hypertension were associated with the presence of carotid plaques. Similar results were found by Ebrahim et al. (1999) in "*The British Regional Heart Study*", which included 425 men and 375 women aged 55 to 76 in two British cities. The authors concluded that increased IMCE and carotid plaques correlated with each other, but showed different patterns of association with cardiovascular risk factors: IMCE measured in the posterior wall of the common carotid artery was associated with risk factors for stroke or previous stroke, on the other hand, IMCE measured at the origin of the bulb (as performed in this study) and the presence of plaques were associated with risk factors for ischemic heart disease or previous diagnosis of the same (Ebrahim et al, 1999). These findings suggest that the pathological processes leading to plaque formation and increased IMT may not be similar and may therefore reflect different aspects of atherogenesis and different clinical manifestations (Jhonsen and Mathiesen, 2009).

B-mode ultrasound was used as the assessment method in this study because it can be easily used to measure arterial stiffness, but its use is limited to the largest and most accessible arteries. Thus, this technique has been used mainly in the brachial, femoral, carotid and abdominal aorta arteries. Several clips and images of the vessel walls can be obtained per cardiac cycle, and the maximum, average and minimum values are calculated by specific *software* on a *workstation*.

The impact of CIMT on the incidence of cardiovascular events in the Rotterdam study, for example, which used B-mode ultrasound CIMT analysis, indicates that the risk of myocardial infarction increases by 43% (Mancini et al, 2004). The main conclusions resulting from this study have been supported by other independent research revealing that CIMT greater than 0.9-1.0 mm indicates potential atherosclerotic disease, which translates into an increased cardiovascular risk (Blaha et al, 2011).

Problems with using ultrasound to assess arterial stiffness include the limited resolution, which can make it difficult to detect very small changes in vessel diameter, the technique also depends heavily on the skill of the operator, as the image of the vessel walls must be studied accurately, so there are concerns about the reproducibility of the technique, which has not yet been very well elucidated, although with an experienced operator, this can be improved.

Although ultrasound has the advantage of being non-invasive when compared to an angiograph, the equipment is expensive, so its use to determine arterial stiffness has largely been confined to the research environment to date (Toth, 2008), but when compared to the value of magnetic resonance equipment, the cost-benefit is well worth it, even though magnetic resonance has much higher spatial resolution.

Chapter 2

2.   BACKGROUND

Few data are available in the medical literature to support and describe the prognostic value of CIMT in patients surviving an acute coronary event.

A few years ago, the International Atherosclerosis Project (Robertson, 1967) already indicated that the process of subclinical atherosclerosis occurs simultaneously in the carotid, coronary and cerebral beds, which justifies our interest in investigating their respective outcomes in these patients, In addition, evidence has shown that generalized atherosclerosis is also reflected by carotid atherosclerosis, which is accurately detected by ultrasound, even in B-mode, which is feasible and has a high degree of reproducibility in estimating CIMT.

Through the ERICO study we will have the opportunity to introduce the possibility of an early diagnosis of subclinical carotid atherosclerotic disease in patients who have already had an acute coronary event.

For this reason, we evaluated the short- and long-term prognostic value (up to three years of follow-up) in individuals with and without intima-media thickening using the EMIC marker in post-acute coronary syndrome individuals.

Chapter 3

Primary

To evaluate the prognostic value of CIMT in post-acute coronary syndrome patients as a predictor of all-cause mortality, cardiovascular disease and coronary artery disease in the short and long term (180 days, 1.2 and 3 years) in the ERICO study.

Secondary

To evaluate the prognostic value of CIMT in post-acute coronary syndrome patients as a predictor of all-cause mortality, cardiovascular disease and coronary artery disease in the short and long term (180 days, 1, 2 and 3 years) stratified by age (<65 years and >65 years) in the ERICO study.

Chapter 4

4.   **METHODS**

4.1 Population and study design

This is a sub-study nested within the ERICO study which aims to assess the prognostic value of atherosclerosis in the carotid arteries using CME in post-ACS individuals.

All the participants in the ERICO project were included in this study and underwent the following procedures 30 days after the acute event: collection of laboratory tests, blood pressure measurement, and imaging tests such as ultrasound of the carotid arteries to check the MIS.

4.2 Study of the Acute Coronary Syndrome Registry Strategy - ERICO

The ERICO study is an ongoing prospective cohort study involving all consecutive cases of ACS treated at HU-USP from February 2009 to December 2013. HU-USP is a medium-complexity teaching and research unit with 260 beds located in the Butanta district, in the west of the city of Sao Paulo, and is the only public hospital with universal care in the area. It is home to a municipal emergency room, a maternity hospital, 14 basic health units and 4 family health programs.

The Butanta neighborhood had a population of 428,000 in 2010 and a human development index of 0.716 (IBGE, 2010). People living in the HU-USP reference area who come to the hospital because of ACS are treated in the emergency department, the medical ward or a general intensive care unit.

Most patients who need an interventional procedure are referred to the Heart Institute (InCor) of the Hospital das Clínicas of the Faculty of Medicine of the University of São Paulo (HCFMUSP).

4.3 Data collection in the EMIC sub-study of the ERICO study

At hospital admission, all data was collected by trained interviewers with a background in healthcare using standardized questionnaires that obtained sociodemographic data on previous history of CVRF, such as hypertension, diabetes, dyslipidemia, sedentary lifestyle, previous history of coronary heart disease and family history of coronary heart disease. In addition, data was collected on medications used. During hospitalization, all patients were treated at the discretion of the hospital staff. The individuals were re-evaluated by a doctor from the ERICO study 30 days after the acute event, with a new clinical assessment of blood pressure, weight, anthropometric measurements, electrocardiogram, as well as, laboratory evaluations that included the measurement of total cholesterol and its fractions, triglycerides, fasting glucose, hemoglobin A1C, C-reactive protein and a trained and experienced radiology technologist performed an ultrasound of the carotid arteries to check the CME.

After 180 days, and then annually, all subjects were contacted by telephone to update their clinical information, including fatal and non-fatal events during follow-up.

4.4 Definition of acute coronary syndrome

ACS is an umbrella term that encompasses IA, STEMI and STEMI. AMI was defined as the presence of symptoms consistent with cardiac ischemia within 24 hours of hospital presentation and troponin I above the 99th percentile, with a specific coefficient of variation test <10% (Luepker et al, 2003;Thygesen et al, 2007). STEMI was defined as the presence of criteria for AMI plus one of the following: (a) persistent ST-segment elevation of >1 mm in two contiguous electrocardiographic leads, or (b) the presence of a new (or presumed new) bundle branch block. STEMI was defined as the presence of criteria for AMI, but not for STEMI. A diagnosis of IA required the presence of symptoms consistent with cardiac ischemia 24 hours prior to hospital admission, the absence of AMI criteria and at least one of the following events: (a) a history of coronary artery disease (CAD); (B) a positive coronary artery disease stratification test (invasive or non-invasive); (C) transient ST-segment change >0.5 mm in two contiguous leads, new T wave inversion >1 mm and/or pseudonormalization of previously inverted T waves; (D) troponin I >0.4 ng/ml (which guarantees a troponin I level above the 99th percentile, regardless of the kit used); or (e) concordant diagnosis by two independent physicians (Goulart et al, 2013).

4.5 Instruments for evaluating participants

4.5.1   ERICO questionnaire - initial

Patient identification form (Appendix 2) containing: sociodemographic information, personal and family history of risk factors and cardiovascular diseases, information on electrocardiogram and laboratory data at admission, medication, history of current clinical condition, physical examination at admission, diagnosis after initial assessment and final diagnosis (ST-elevation myocardial infarction, non-ST-elevation myocardial infarction, low to high risk angina and other diagnoses not related to ACS).

4.5.2   ERICO Questionnaire - 30 days

Patient identification form (Appendix 3) containing: personal data, vital status, information on recurrence of ACS, stroke, hemodynamic procedures and coronary artery bypass grafting, information on the acute event, medication during the acute event, risk stratification of the acute event, high-dose medication, medication in use, 30-day physical examination.

4.5.3   ERICO questionnaire - 6 months

Patient identification form (Appendix 4) containing: personal data, vital status, information on recurrence of ACS, stroke, medications in use during a 180-day follow-up.

4.5.4   ERICO questionnaire - annual.

Patient identification form (Appendix 4) containing: personal data, vital status, information on recurrence of ACS, stroke, medication in use during a 360-day follow-up.

4.5.5   Laboratory tests

Participants in the ERICO project collected blood and urine samples, which we will use for our research, including: uric acid, total cholesterol, HDL cholesterol, LDL cholesterol, triglycerides, creatinine, urea, glycemic curve (fasting and 120 minutes), glycated hemoglobin and microalbuminuria - isolated urine sample.

4.6 Instruments for assessing carotid intima-media thickness

The EMIC can be measured by ultrasound, where the distance between a double-line reflex pattern representing the lumen-intima and media-adventitia interfaces m the EMIC measurements in histological patterns (Pignoli et al, 1986).

Images of the carotid arteries were acquired and analyzed by an experienced radiology technologist according to the protocol previously defined in the Longitudinal Study of Adult Health (ELSA-Brazil) (Trichopoulou et al, 2003; Willett et al, 1995) and the data was recorded in an individual table for each participant (Appendix 5). EMIC was assessed in all subjects who took part in the personal interview 30 days after the acute event, in a standardized manner, using B-mode ultrasound equipment (Aplio XG™, Toshiba). Images of the bilateral carotid artery were taken using a linear ultrasound transducer type SSA-770A (Toshiba, Tokyo, Japan) with an average frequency of 7.5 MHz (ranging from 5-11 MHz in frequency).

4.6.1   Anatomy of the carotid artery complex

The cervical carotid arteries are the largest caliber arteries in the cervical region. The right CCA originates from the innominate artery and the left CCA originates directly from the aortic arch. The cervical carotid arteries are ascending, lateral and posterior to the trachea. In the plane of the thyroid cartilage, slightly below the angle of the mandible, the common carotid bifurcates into the external and internal carotids. Proximal to the bifurcation, the right common carotid dilates to form the carotid bulb. The origin of the bulb can be recognized in most individuals. It is defined as the place where the carotid artery begins to dilate and the vessel walls curve laterally, no longer parallel to the skin surface. The bulb has an elliptical morphology and complex geometry in the longitudinal axis. Its cranial limit is defined as the flow divider point. The tip of the flow divider is also an anatomical reference for the origin of the internal and external carotid arteries. The external carotid artery courses anteriorly and slightly medially to the internal carotid artery in 90% of individuals. The remaining 10% have an inverse orientation. The external carotid is generally smaller in caliber than the internal carotid and has branches that supply the neck and face. The internal carotid has no cervical branches and travels upwards to the brain (Oliveira et al, 2008).

4.6.2 Anatomy of interest

The extracranial carotid arteries were assessed bilaterally, in the distal segment of the common carotid artery. No images were taken of the external and internal carotid arteries, as the associations do not have the same patterns for the common carotid artery and the internal carotid artery, because the reproducibility of the study of the internal carotid artery is low in local and international experience.

Anatomical definitions: the distal common carotid is the segment of the common carotid immediately proximal to the origin of the carotid bulb, where the proximal and distal walls are parallel to each other. The end of the common carotid is demarcated by the dilation of the vessel walls, forming the carotid bulb.

4.6.3 Participant's position for image acquisition

The radiology technologist positioned the subject in the supine position during the carotid scan, so as to allow him to turn his head sideways. The radiology technologist then attached three ECG clips for simultaneous acquisition of the image and cardiac cycles, in the following sequence:

1. green clip - on the ankle of one of the lower limbs;
2. red clip - on the right upper limb cuff;
3. yellow clip - on the cuff of the left upper limb.

The examiner then sits or stands next to the diva, close to the individual's head. The head is placed at 45° in the opposite direction to the side being examined. Subjects were instructed not to turn their head to look at the equipment's monitor screen. The individual's head was positioned by the sonographer at the beginning of the study, while asking the individual not to swallow or move during the examination.

The study began on the left side, according to protocol.

The transducer was positioned longitudinally between the anterior and posterior trigone of the neck, so that the position of the transducer may be above the sternocleidomastoid muscle, adjusting the acoustic window so that the inside of the vessel shows only a few sparse echoes.

4.6.4 Initial examination (clip)

The sonographer scanned in the transverse axis, starting in the plane of the carotid bifurcation (in the plane of the mandible angle), including the carotid bulb and ending in the distal segment of the common carotid artery. The aim of the initial examination was to guide the sonographer in relation to the anatomical path of the segments of interest in the individual's carotid territory.

4.6.5 Image documentation protocol

A sequence of scans in the transverse axis was recorded, lasting 8 seconds. Next, the image of the distal common carotid artery was taken in the longitudinal axis, with a 10-mm extension, measured from the beginning of the bulb, and recorded dynamically, simultaneously with the ECG spectrum. This recording lasted 3 heartbeat cycles.

The image of the distal common carotid artery was taken at a depth of 4 cm, *pre-set* in the equipment's "*pre-set*" and kept constant throughout the exam, on both sides. In short, the sonographer recorded:

1.Clip of the transverse scan of the common carotid, in the transverse axis, from the carotid bifurcation to the distal common carotid, including the bulb, lasting 8 seconds.

2Image clip of the distal common carotid artery (1O-mm distal), in the longitudinal axis, coupled to the spectral trace of the ECG, with a duration of 3 cardiac cycles.

In this clip, the carotid bulb should be to the left of the monitor. If the bulb has not been identified, the tip of the flow divider can be used as an anatomical repair. After locating the tip of the flow divider and centering its image on the screen, the transducer should be moved to the lateral plane of the neck and moved caudally. Next, the transducer is centered on the distal segment of the common carotid, just bulbar, 1Omm from the bulb. The transducer should be angled at around 45 degrees so that the best image of the intima-media layer of the common carotid artery, on the posterior wall, is obtained, as this is generally the best angle of incidence for obtaining an optimal image of the common carotid artery (Oliveira et al, 2OO8).

4.6.6   Satisfactory image criteria

The criterion for satisfactory B-mode ultrasound images of the carotid arteries is defined as the clear visualization of the interfaces of the arterial walls in the longitudinal axis and of the arterial anatomical repairs.

Distal wall - arterial wall furthest from the transducer lumen - intima interface and media - adventitia interface.

The area of interest was positioned in the center of the image. The transducer was aligned to show as much of the vessel as possible in the cranio-caudal axis. The sonographer should optimize the visualization of the arterial interfaces by adjusting the overall gain or by pressing the *Quick Sean* key (gain adjustment).

automatic), the direction of the sound beam and the positioning of the transducer.

In order to obtain a clear image of the intimal layer of the common carotid artery, the gain setting needs to be high compared to conventional clinical studies. Thus, a satisfactory ultrasound image of the carotid lumen is expected to contain a minimal amount of artifacts.

Satisfactory images were obtained at a standardized depth, which should, in principle, be kept the same for all longitudinal shots.

The layers of the carotid walls should be demonstrated using high-resolution ultrasound images. In longitudinal sections of the carotid arteries, these layers are visualized as two parallel echogenic lines, separated by a hypoechogenic layer. The arterial walls are best seen in the common carotid, where the vessel runs parallel to the skin surface, thus representing an area situated at a right angle (90°) to the insonation beam.

The first echo along the distal wall of the common carotid artery is derived from the lumen-intima interface and the second echo, usually brighter, originates from the media-adventitia interface. Between these interfaces lies the middle layer, which appears as a hypoechogenic zone. The distance between the first two lines corresponds to the sum of the thickness of the intima and media. Due to its collagen content, the adventitia is hyperechogenic and appears as a shiny zone highlighted at its inner margin by the middle layer. In turn, the periadventitia, depending on its location, is composed of loose areolar tissue and in most cases is hypoechogenic.

Thickening of the intima-media layer is the first abnormality that can be categorically identified on B-mode US. The progression of atherosclerotic disease is associated with increased technical limitations in the process of morphological assessment of vascular lesions, as a result of the
posterior acoustic shadowing present in larger lesions.

Documentation of the posterior wall of the common carotid artery, in its distal segment, should be prioritized. When atherosclerotic lesions are identified in the distal segment and/or the carotid bulb (Oliveira et al, 2008).

4.6.7   Image analysis

After acquisition, the EMIC images were sent to a workstation for reading in specific software (*Carotid Analyzer for Research - Medical Imaging Analyzer, MIA™*), and the measurements provided for in the protocol of the Longitudinal Study of Adult Health (ELSA-Brazil) were taken. The *workstation* system makes it possible to analyze the images using specific *software.*

The first step in analyzing carotid images is calibration. The equipment is set up so that the study is carried out with a fixed calibration. The reader assumes that the magnification level does not change during the EMIC assessment.

The measurements taken on the images of the carotid arteries were made using the lines demarcated by the *software* on the proximal and distal walls. The lines were marked on the common carotid artery, about 10 meters long, proximal to the carotid bulb. The EMIC will only be measured on the image of the posterior wall of the distal segment of the common carotid artery. For an experienced image reader, the task of tracing the lines on a good quality image of a normal artery is relatively simple. Measurements of vessel caliber, vascular lumen and EMIC in the distal wall were obtained during 3 cardiac cycles. The *software*'s measurement algorithm calculates the distance between the lines delimiting the anatomical structures of the vessels and issues a report of the minimum, maximum and average values (with standard deviation). The anatomical structures of the vascular wall are defined by pairs of lines (Oliveira et al, 2008).

EMIC was measured in the common carotid artery on the right and left sides. EMIC was defined as the mean values obtained in the right and left common carotid arteries (avg-avg EMIC). We observed EMIC in both the proximal and distal walls, but due to physical sonographic factors, we decided to use only the value for the distal wall. Images of the common carotid arteries were acquired over a length of 4 cm, including the carotid bifurcation (on the left side of the screen) and the distal tergus of the common carotid artery. A measurement point of 1 cm below the carotid bifurcation was assumed, analyzing the distal segment of the common carotid artery, before the carotid bifurcation, regardless of the presence of plaques.

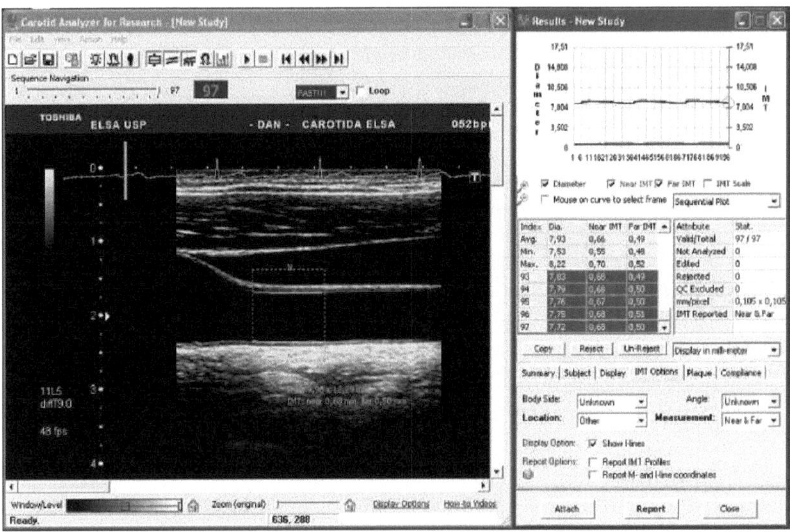

Figure 1 - Location of the EMIC measurement in the *Carotid Analyzer for Research - Medical Imaging Analyzer,* MIA™ software.

4.6.8   Image quality classification ("*Score*")

The criterion for satisfactory image quality was defined according to the protocol established in the ELSA cohort (Oliveira, 2008).

Although the "*score*" is subjective, below are some standards to guide the classification of the quality of images of both healthy and diseased arteries.

- Unacceptable: 0 or demarcated line.
- Poor: 2 lines, a pair, drawn, resulting in the measurement of the lumen or caliber of the vessel.
    - Acceptable: 2 or 3 lines with two measurements of the expected tres (EMI and lumen).
    - Very good: all 6 lines marked out, all three measurements taken.
    - Excellent: the six lines clearly visualized and demarcated, with good image quality and positioning (Oliveira et al, 2008).

This analysis depended on the number of lines that were displayed, the lines that define the proximal (adventitia-media, intima-media, intima-blood) and distal (intima-blood, intima-media and media-adventitia) wall interfaces. This process of image acquisition and EMIC measurement was carried out by an experienced radiology technologist trained specifically for this function and analyzed by radiologists at the Clinical and Epidemiological Research Center (CPCE) which is centralized in the ultrasound reading center of the ELSA-Brazil cohort, located in Sao Paulo, Brazil.

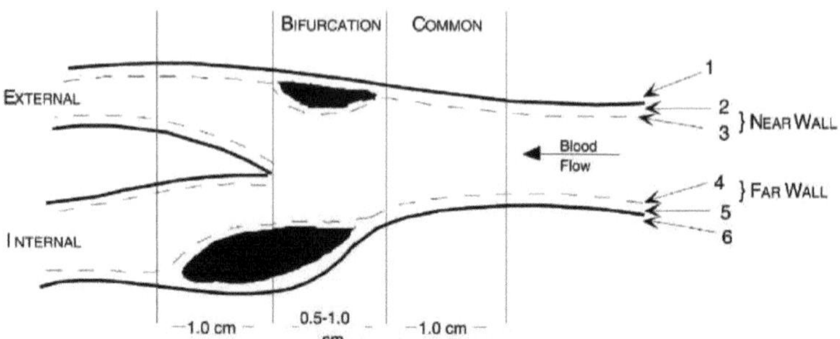

Figure 2 - Schematic lines representing the interfaces of the carotid artery on ultrasound.

4.7 Definition of general and specific mortality

In this study, mortality was analyzed for all causes, cardiovascular disease and coronary artery disease. Participants were defined as having a cardiovascular cause of death when they identified a cause of death classified in version 10 of the International Classification of Diseases (ICD 10) Chapter IX "Diseases of the circulatory system" or if they identified a cause of death classified with ICD-10 code R57.0 "Cardiogenic shock." (QMS, 2010).

Vital status was investigated periodically using an active strategy involving telephone searches and medical records from HU-USP during follow-up. Mortality data was confirmed by official death certificates with the collaboration of the municipality (Programa de Aprimoramento das Informações de Mortalidade sem Municipio de Sao Paulo, PRO-AIM), the state (Fundaçao Sistema Estadual de Análise de Dados-SEADE) and the Ministry of Health.

4.8 Ethics

An informed consent form was obtained from all participants with potential signs and symptoms of ACS or their legal guardian on admission to hospital, once they had agreed to take part in the study (Appendix 1).

The research protocol was approved by the Research Ethics Committee of HU-USP under registration number CEP HU-USP 1565/16 (APPENDIX 1).

4.9 Statistical analysis

Baseline characteristics, FRCV and ACS subtypes were compared according to the EMIC tertiles, which was presented as a combined measure of the mean value between the averages generated from the right and left common carotid artery (med-med).

Continuous variables were tested for normal distribution using the Kolmogorov-Smirnov test and, as long as most of them had a non-parametric distribution, they were presented as medians with the respective interquartile ranges. The Kruskal-Wallis test was used for continuous variables. Categorical variables were presented as absolute and relative frequencies tested using the chi-square test.

Case fatality rates at 180 days, 1, 2 and 3 years were also compared according to EMIC tertiles. In addition, survival analyses were carried out up to 1, 2 and 3 years of follow-up, considering all-cause mortality, CVD mortality and CAD mortality, using Kaplan-Meier survival curve analysis with the *log-rank* test and

Cox proportional hazards models to calculate risk ratios (RR) with respective 95% confidence intervals (95% CI). All RRs were calculated crudely, adjusted for age, age-sex and finally multivariate adjustment was carried out which additionally included education (no formal education, elementary school, high school and college), hypertension (yes or no), diabetes (yes or no) and dyslipidemia (yes or no) and smoking (current, past and never). Additional adjustments for race and ACS subtype were also tested in the multivariate models.

Survival analyses stratified by age (<65 years and > 65 years) were also carried out.

A sensitivity analysis was carried out excluding individuals with an EMIC greater than 1.5 mm (78 individuals), which may correspond to carotid plaque (Touboul et al, 2007; Touboul et al, 2011).

For all analyses, P values of less than 0.05 were considered significant. All statistical analyses were carried out using SPSS *software* version 24.0 and the R statistical program.

Chapter 5

5. RESULTS

5.1 Casuistry

Of the 1085 participants included in the ERICO study, a total of 718 (66.17%) participants had complete EMIC data acquired 30 days after an acute event. Of these 718 participants, 653 (90.9%) had complete and good quality EMIC data acquired 30 days after the ACS event. Nine (1.25%) individuals who reported being of Asian or indigenous origin were excluded, giving a total of 644 (89.7%) study participants. Although this approach could adjust for race/ethnicity effects, it was not possible to study each of these ethnic minority groups due to the smaller number of participants in each stratum in the ERICO study.

5.2 Sociodemographic characteristics, cardiovascular risk factors and ACS subtypes.

Among the 644 cases of EMIC evaluated in this sample with a median age of 61 years (interquartile range (IQR): 52-71 years), 400 participants were under 65 years of age. The median EMIC was 0.74 mm ± 0.20 (IQR: 0.40- 1.90 millimeters). Most of the participants analyzed were male (61.7%), white (66.9%), married (62.9%) and with a low level of education (61.8%). The most common cardiovascular risk factors found were obesity (75.6%) followed by hypertension (75.2%), a sedentary lifestyle (67.7%), dyslipidemia (45%), diabetes (36%), smoking (31.3%) and a previous history of CHD (25.0%). The proportion of ACS subtypes was 29.7% angina, 39.9% STEMI and 30.4% STEMI. Age, hypertension, diabetes and dyslipidemia, as well as a lower level of education were all associated with higher EMIC values. Other CVRFs or ACS subtypes were not statistically associated with EMIC (table 1).

Table 1. Baseline characteristics of the 644 participants in the ERICO cohort according to EMIC tertiles, 2009-2013.

Sociodemographic characteristics	1° (n= 212)	2° (n= 220)	3° (n= 212)	Total	P-value
EMIC tercis					
Men (%)	124 (58.5)	144 (65.5)	129 (60.8)	397 (61.65)	0.32
Median age, years (IQR)	54 (47-62)	63(55-71)	66 (59-75)		<0.001
Raga (%)					
White	138 (65.1)	149 (67.7)	144 (67.9)	431 (66.92)	n
Brown	59 (27.8)	60 (27.3)	60 (28.3)	179 (27.80)	x. 66

Black	15(7.1)	11 (5.0)	8 (3,8)	34 (5.28)	
Marital status (%)					
Single	33 (15.6)	33 (15.0)	26(12.3)	92 (14.29)	
Married	137(64.6)	141 (64.1)	127 (60.2)	405 (62.89)	0.
Divorced	20 (9.4)	16(7.3)	14 (6.6)	50 (7.76)	10
Widowed	22(10.4)	30 (13.6)	44 (20.9)	96(14.90)	

Education (%)					
No formal education	19(9.0)	24(10.9)	31 (14.6)	74(11.49)	
Elementary school	123 (58.0)	134(60.9)	141 (66.5)	398 (61.80)	0.
High school	45 (21.2)	40 (18.2)	29(13.7)	114(17.70)	04
Higher education	25 (11.8)	22 (10.0)	H(5.2)	58 (9.01)	
Cardiovascular risk factors					

Smoking (%)					
Current	73 (35.1)	68 (31.8)	55 (26.8)	196 (31.26)	n
Past	70 (33.7)	82 (38.3)	87 (42.4)	239 (38.12)	χ^2 35
Never	65 (31.3)	64 (29.9)	63 (30.7)	192 (30.62)	
Median BMI, kg/m^2 (IQR)	27.10 (24.3-30.0)	26.05 (23.7-29.6)	26.6 (24.1-30.1)		0.22
Obesity (%)	158 (74.5)	170 (77.3)	159 (75.0)	487 (75.62)	0.78

Hypertension (%)	142 (67.9)	161 (75.2)	173 (82.4)	476 (73.91)	0.003

Continuaba©...

Diabetes (%)	61(28.9)	74 (34.7)	97 (46.6)	232 (36.02)	0.001
Dyslipidemia (%)	96 (48.2)	84 (44.4)	110(59.1)	290 (45.03)	0.01
Heart failure (%)	33 (16.9)	32 (16.4)	35 (19.4)	100 (15.53)	0.71
AVE (%)	15 (7.4)	20 (9.8)	23 (11.9)	58 (9.01)	0.30
Sedentary lifestyle (%)	148 (72.2)	146 (69.5)	142 (70.6)	436 (67.70)	0.84
Previous history of CHD (%)	55 (27.5)	47 (22.6)	49 (25.0)	151 (23.45)	0.52
Subtypes of ACS					

Unstable angina	66 (31.1)	64 (29.1)	61 (28.8)	191 (29.66)
IAMSSST	80 (37.7)	85 (38.6)	92 (43.4)	257 (39.91)
IAMCSST	66 (31.1)	71 (32.3)	59 (27.8)	196 (30.43)

(P Value: 0.74)

EMIC values: 1st tertile (0.40-0.70 mm), 2nd tertile (0.71-0.80 mm) and 3rd tertile (0.81-1.90 mm).
Some proportions may not add up to 100° due to rounding or falling values (maximum 8.85° in
heart failure). P values were obtained using the Chi-square test for categorical variables and the Kruskal-Wallis test for continuous variables.
IQR: interquartile range. BMI: body mass index. CVA: cerebrovascular accident. CHD: coronary heart disease. ACS: acute coronary syndrome.
STEMI: acute myocardial infarction without ST-segment elevation. STEMI: acute myocardial infarction with ST-segment elevation.

In relation to the association of EMIC with lipids, we found a slight increase in HDL levels after the acute phase of the coronary event in the 3rd° tertile of EMIC (Table 2).

Table 2. Lipid profile of the ERICO cohort according to EMIC tertiles, 2009-2013.

Features	EMIC med-med			P Value
Acute phase (24-48 hours after ACS)	1st tertile	2° tertile	3° tertile	
Lipid variables				

Total cholesterol, mg/dl	180 (146-209)	173 (143-204)	170 (143-215)	0,83
LDL-cholesterol, mg/dl	103 (79-133)	107 (81-133)	101 (79-138)	0.92
HDL-cholesterol, mg/dl	37 (30-43)	37 (32-46)	38 (32-46)	0.41
HDL-cholesterol ratio	4.72 (3.77-5.66)	4.44 (3.67-5.45)	4.73 (3.88-5.66)	0.41
TC:HDL cholesterol ratio	4.74 (3.80-5.68)	4.49 (3.67-5.50)	4.71 (3.88-5.66)	0.50
Triglycerides, mg/dl	130(97-190)	133 (100-175)	135.50 (102.5-194.5)	0.62
Subacute phase (30-45 days after ACS)				
Total cholesterol, mg/dl				

LDL-cholesterol, mg/dl	145 (124-168)	144(122-175)	150 (127-185)	0.30
HDL-cholesterol, mg/dl	77 (61.5-93.5)	81.5 (58-98.25)	83 (66-103)	0.18
Total cholesterol, mg/dl	37 (32-44)	39.5 (31.75-48)	41 (35-48)"	0.008
TC:HDL ratio	3.85 (3.28-4.5)	3.70 (3.15-4.31)	3.78 (3.07-4.40)	0.25
Triglycerides, mg/dl	129 (96-188)	123.5 (94,75-162.5)	124 (93-165)	0.35

Lipids are presented in median and interquartile ranges (IQR). P values were obtained from Kruskal-Wallis.
* P-value <0.001 comparing dead and alive participants.
** P-value <0.05 comparing dead participants
and alive. ACS: acute coronary syndrome.

5.3 Global lethality rates

During three years of follow-up, there were 65 deaths (10.1%), and the lethality rates were progressively higher among the EMIC tertiles in all periods, with the highest rates being observed in participants with the highest EMIC (3° tertile) (180 days: 6.6% vs. 1 year: 9.0% vs. 2 years: 12.3% vs. 3 years: 16.0%, P <0.05) (Table 3). When the analysis was stratified by age, <65 years and >65 years, we found P<0.05 only at the 180-day follow-up (Table 3).

Table 3. Case-fatality rates at 180 days, 1 year, 2 years and 3 years in the ERICO cohort according to EMIC tertiles, 2009-2013.

	180 days	1 year	2 years	3 years

General (n=644)				
EMIC **1°** (0.40-0.70 mm)	4/212 (1.9)**	5/212 (2.4)**	8/212(3.8)**	11/212(5.2)*
2° (0.71-0.80 mm)	4/220 (1.8)**	9/220 (4.1)**	13/220 (5.9)**	20/220 (9.1)*
3° (0.81-1.9 mm)	14/212(6.6)**	19/212(9.0)**	26/212 (12.3)**	34/212 (16.0)*
< 65 years(n=400)				
EMIC **1°** (0.40-0.70 mm)	1/122 (0.8)**	2/122 (1.6)	3/122 (2.5)	4/122 (3.6)
2° (0.71-0.80 mm)	0/143 (0.0)**	1/143 (0.7)	3/143 (2.1)	6/143 (4.2)
3° (0.81-1.9 mm)	5/135(3.7)**	6/135 (4.4)	8/135 (5.9)	10/135 (7.4)

> 65 years(n=244)				
EMIC **1°** (0.40-0.70 mm)	5/84 (6.0)	9/84 (10.7)	12/84(14.3)	17/84 (20.2)
2° (0.71-0.80 mm)	2/82 (2.4)	4/82 (4.9)	9/82(11.0)	13/82 (15.9)
3° (0.81-1.9 mm)	9/78 (11.5)	11/78 (14.1)	12/78 (15.4)	15/78 (19.2)

Lethality rates are the proportion of the population that died / total at risk) (° o) P values were obtained from the Chi-square test.

* P-value <0.001 comparing dead and alive participants.

** P-value <0.05 comparing dead and alive participants.

5.4 All-cause survival, CVD and CAD

Lower survival rates were observed for all-cause mortality, CVD and CAD according to EMIC tertiles.

For all-cause mortality, survival estimates in days were inversely associated with EMIC tertiles (2,182 days for the 1st° vs. 2,051 days for the 2nd vs. 1,817 days for the 30th, *p-Log Rank* <0.001), as shown in figure 3.

Figure 3 Kaplan-Meier survival curve for all-cause mortality by EMIC tertiles at up to three years of follow-up among ACS patients in the ERICO cohort, 2009-2013.

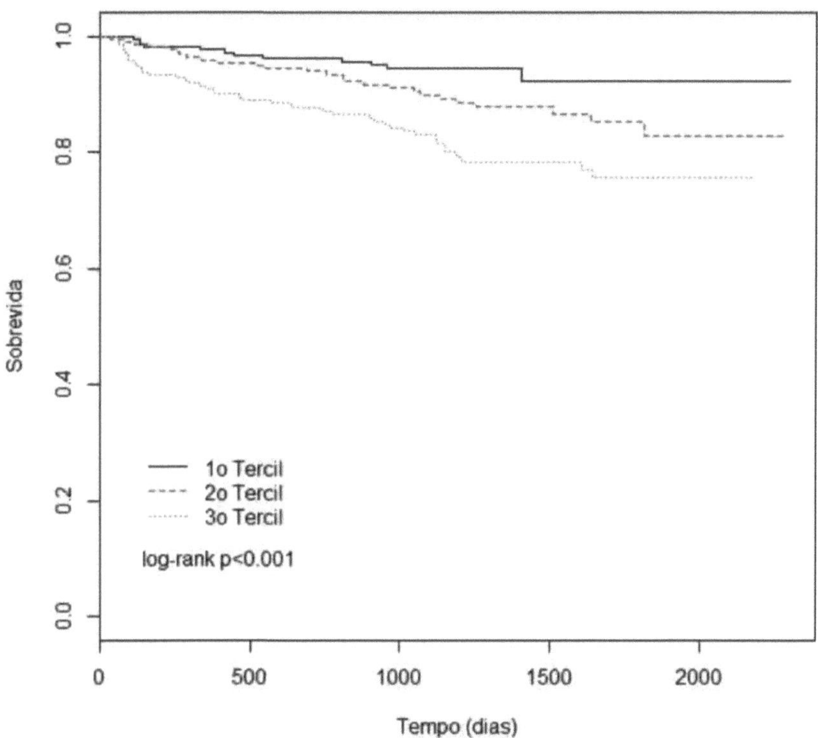

Mean survival time (95% CI) according to all-cause mortality by EMIC tertiles

Tercis IMT	Events/Individuals	Censored cases	Average time		
				95% CI	
			Media(days)	Lower limit	Upper limit
1° (0.40-0.70 mm)	212/13	199 (93.9%)	2.182	2.118	2.246
2° (0.71-0.80 mm)	220/26	194 (88.2%)	2.051	1.969	2.133
3° (0.81-1.9 mm)	212/42	170 (80.2%)	1.817	1.719	1.915
Total	644/81	563 (87.4%)	2.052	2.001	2.104

For CVD mortality, survival estimates in days were also inversely associated with EMIC tertiles (2,246 days for I° tertile vs. 2,140 days for the 2nd tertile *vs.* 1,962 days for the 30th, *p-Log Rank* = 0.003), as shown in figure 4.

Figure 4 Kaplan-Meier survival curve for cardiovascular disease mortality by EMIC tertiles at up to three years of follow-up among ACS patients in the ERICO cohort, 2009-2013.

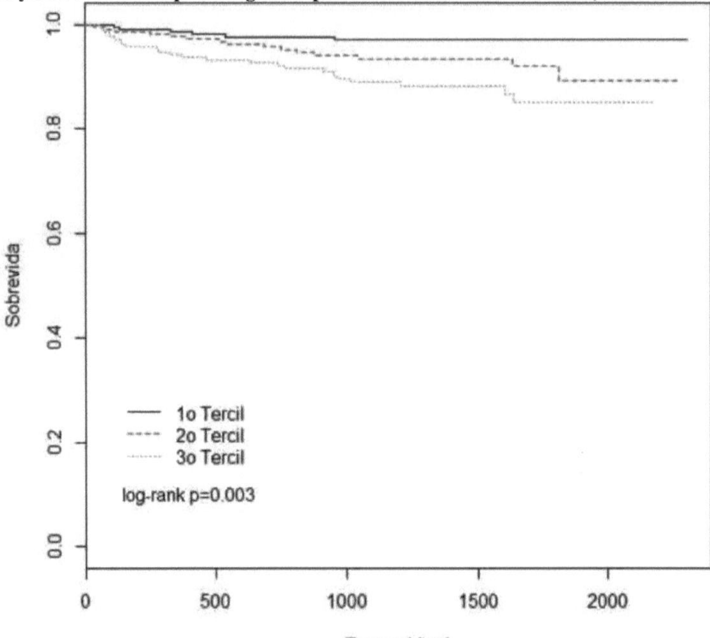

Mean survival time (95% CI) according to mortality from cardiovascular disease by tertiles of the

Tercis IMT	EMIC		Average time		
	Events/Individuals	Censored cases	Average (days)	95% CI	
				Lower limit	Upper limit
1° (0.40-0.70 mm)	212/6	206 (97.2%)	2.246	2.202	2.291
2° (0.71-0.80 mm)	220/15	205 (93.2%)	2.140	2.072	2.208
3° (0.81-1.9 mm)	212/24	188 (88.7%)	1.962	1.881	2.043
Total	644/45	599 (93.0%)	2.158	2.117	2.199

For mortality from CAD, we found greater differences in average survival in days between the 1st° tercile: 2,293 days compared to the other two tertiles (2nd tercile: 2,181 days and 3rd tercile: 2,075 *days, p-LogRank* = 0.0015), as shown in figure 5.

Figure 5 Kaplan-Meier survival curve for mortality from coronary artery disease by EMIC tertiles at up to three years of follow-up among ACS patients in the ERICO cohort, 2009-2013.

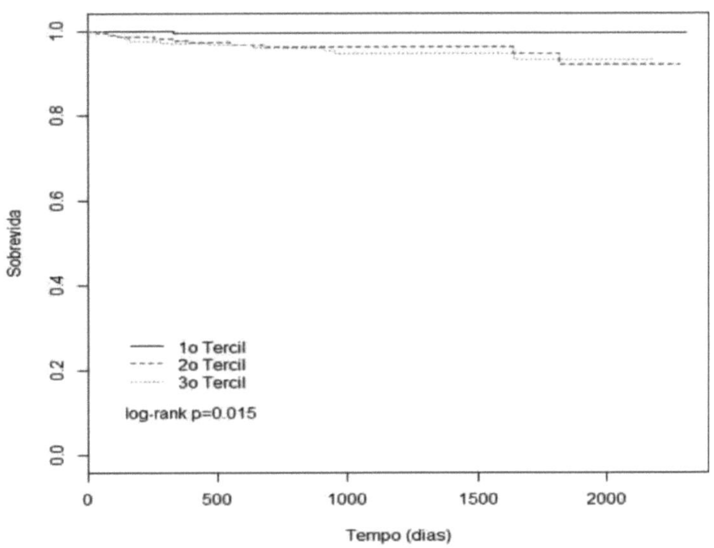

Mean survival time (95% CI) according to mortality from coronary artery disease by EMIC tertiles					
	Media time				
Tercis IMT	Events/Individuals	Censored cases	Average (days)	95% CI	
				Lower limit	Upper limit
1° (0.40-0.70 mm)	212/1	211 (99.5%)	2.293	2.275	2.312
2° (0.71-0.80 mm)	220/10	205 (95.5%)	2.181	2.121	2.240
3° (0.81-1.9 mm)	212/11	201 (94.8%)	2.075	2.016	2.134
Total	644/22	622 (96.6%)	2.228	2.197	2.259

Of the 65 deaths in the sample, 45 (69.2%) were due to cardiovascular disease and 22 (33.8%) had coronary artery disease as the main cause of death during the 3-year follow-up.

In the overall COX analysis, we found higher risk ratios (RR) for death from all causes and CVD from 1 to 3 years and for CAD only at 2 and 3 years. However, no significant results remained after adjusting for age and other confounding factors such as gender, education and CVRF (Tables 4, 5 and 6).

Adjustments for race and ACS subtype did not change the results.

Table 4: Risk ratio (RR) [95% confidence interval (CI)] of all-cause mortality in participants of the ERICO cohort according to EMIC tertiles, 2009-2013.

All causes	1 year Risk ratio CI 5th/$_{90}$	2 years Risk ratio CI 5th/$_{90}$	3 years Risk ratio CI 0$_{95}$/$_0$
No adjustment			
1st tertile	Reference (1,00)	Reference (1,00)	Reference (1,00)
2nd tertile	1.96 (0.67-5.74)	1.61 (0.66-3.87)	1.78 (0.85-3.72)
3rd tertile	3.97 (1.48-10.64)	3.42 (1.55-7.55)	3.25 (1.65-6.41)
Age adjustment			

1st tertile	Reference (1,00)	Reference (1,00)	Reference (1,00)
2nd tertile	1.15 (0.38-3.48)	0.96 (0.39-2.38)	1.09 (0.51-2.34)
3rd tertile	1.92 (0.67-5.49)	1.71 (0.73-4.00)	1.70 (0.82-3.50)
Adjustment by age and gender			
1st tertile	Reference (1,00)	Reference (1,00)	Reference (1,00)
2nd tertile	1.14(0.38-3.46)	0.96 (0.38-2.39)	1.10(0.51-2.37)
3rd tertile	1.91 (0.68-5.46)	1.71 (0.73-4.00)	1.71 (0.82-3.54)
Multivariate adjustment			

1st tertile	Reference (1,00)	Reference (1,00)	Reference (1,00)
2nd tertile	0.91 (0.28-2,91)	3.06 (0.31-29.74)	1.10 (0.35-3.50)
3rd tertile	1.54 (0.53-4.44)	3.37 (0.36-31.70)	1.58 (0.54-4.63)

1st tertile :0.40-0.70 mm, 2nd tertile :0.71-0.80 mm and 3rd tertile >0.81 mm.

Multivariate adjustment: age, gender, education, hypertension, diabetes, dyslipidemia and smoking.

Table 5: Risk ratio (RR) [95% confidence interval (CI)] of mortality from cardiovascular diseases in participants in the ERICO cohort according to EMIC tertiles, 2009-2013.

Cardiovascular Diseases	1 year Risk ratio CI 5th/90	2 years Risk ratio CI 5th/90	3 years Risk ratio CI 095/o
No adjustment			
1st tertile	Reference (1,00)	Reference (1,00)	Reference (1,00)
2° tertile	1.63 (0.39-6.84)	1.78 (.060-5.31)	2.13 (0.81-5.59)
3° tertile	4.18 (1.18-14.81)	3.16 (1.15-8.70)	3.68 (1.49-9.12)
Age adjustment			
1st tertile	Reference (1,00)	Reference (1,00)	Reference (1,00)
2° tertile	1.04 (0.24-4.53)	1.15 (0.37-3.56)	1.35 (0.50-3.65)
3° tertile	2.26 (0.59-8.70)	1.75 (0.59-5.18)	2.00 (0.76-5.24)
Adjustment by age and gender			

1st tertile	Reference (1,00)	Reference (1,00)	Reference (1,00)
2° tertile	1.05 (0.24-4.62)	1.15 (0.37-3.56)	1.36(0.50-3.69)
3° tertile	2.28 (0.59-8.81)	1.75 (0.59-5.18)	2.01 (0.77-5.29)
Multivariate adjustment			
1st tertile	Reference (1,00)	Reference (1,00)	Reference (1,00)
2° tertile	0.91 (0.19-4.28)	0.93 (0.37-2.35)	1.43 (0.52-3.95)
3° tertile	1.87(0.49-7.15)	1.46 (0.62-3.44)	2.83 (0.69-4.85)
1st tertile: 0.40-0.70 mm, 2° tertile :0.71-0.80 mm and 3° tercile >0.81 mm.			
Multivariate adjustment: age, gender, education, hypertension, diabetes, dyslipidemia and smoking.			

Table 6. Risk Ratio (RR) [95% Confidence Interval (CI)] of mortality from coronary artery disease in participants of the ERICO cohort according to EMIC tertiles, 2009-2013.

Coronary Artery Disease	1 year Risk ratio CI 5th/$_{90}$	2 years Risk ratio CI 5th/$_{90}$	3 years Risk ratio CI $_{095/0}$
No adjustment			
1st tertile	Reference (1,00)	Reference (1,00)	Reference (1,00)
2° tertile	4.90 (0.57-41.93)	6.92 (0.85-56.23)	7.87 (0.98-62.93)
3° tertile	6.26 (0.75-51.99)	8.41 (1.05-67.24)	10.50(1.34-82.02)
Age adjustment			
1st tertile	Reference (1,00)	Reference (1,00)	Reference (1,00)
2° tertile	3.75 (0.42-33.57)	5.12(0.61-43.11)	6.16 (0.75-50.80)
3° tertile	4.34(0.48-39.28)	5.60 (0.65-47.78)	7.56 (0.92-62.37)

	Adjustment by age and gender		
1st tertile	Reference (1,00)	Reference (1,00)	Reference (1,00)
2° tertile	3.62 (0.40-32.57)	4.87(0.58-41.26)	6.09 (0.74-50.34)
3° tertile	4.22 (0.46-38.29)	5.38 (0.63-46.06)	7.48 (0.90-61.86)
Multivariate adjustment			
1st tertile	Reference (1,00)	Reference (1,00)	Reference (1,00)
2° tertile	3.06 (0.31-29.74)	4.80 (0.55-41.94)	6.80 (0.80-54.56)
3° tertile	3.37 (0.36-31.70)	5.15 (0.59-44.76)	7.17 (0.84-60.83)

1°tercile :0.40-0.70 mm, 2°tercile :0.71-0.80 m and 3°tercile >0.81 mm.
Multivariate adjustment: age, gender, education, hypertension, diabetes, dyslipidemia and smoking.

In the analysis stratified by age, in the group aged <65 years, there was no statistically significant difference for all-cause mortality in the estimates of survival in days (*p-Log Rank* = 0.457), as shown in figure 6.

Figure 6 Kaplan-Meier survival curve for all-cause mortality by EMIC tertiles at up to three years of follow-up among individuals aged less than 65 years with ACS in the ERICO cohort, 2009-2013.

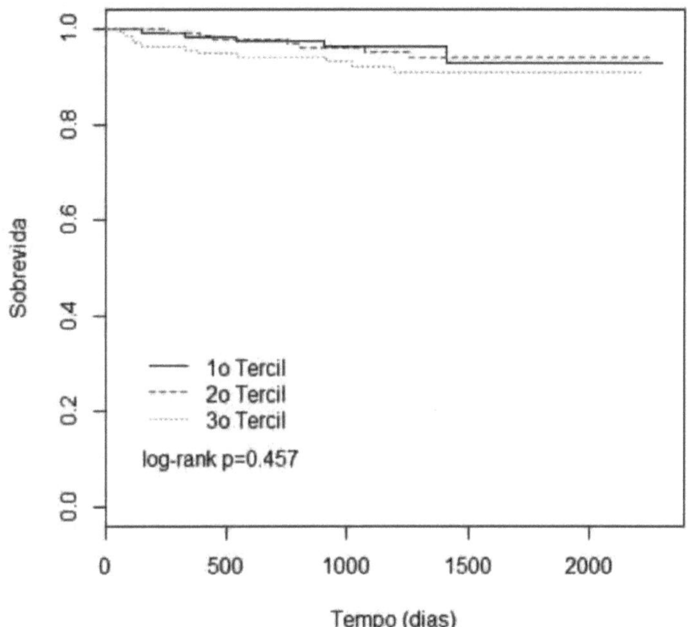

Mean survival time (95% CI) according to EMIC tertiles in individuals under 65 years of age

Tercis IMT (< 65 years)	Events/Individuals	Censored cases	Average (days)	Media (Time) 95% CI	
				Lower limit	Upper limit
1° (0.40-0.60 mm)	122/6	116(95.1%)	2.208	2.134	2.282
2° (0.61-0.80 mm)	143/7	136 (95.1%)	2.157	2.091	2.222
3° (0.81-1.50 mm)	135/11	124 (91.9%)	2.069	1.979	2.158

| Total | 400/24 | 376 (94.0%) | 2.185 | 2.140 | 2.231 |

In the analysis stratified by age, in the group aged <65 years, for CVD mortality, the survival estimates in days were inversely associated with the tertiles of the EMIC (2,271 days for the 1st° tertile vs. *2,206* days for the 2nd° tertile *vs.* 2,095 days for the *3rd, p- LogRank* = 0.047), as shown in figure 7. **Figure 7. Kaplan-Meier survival curve for cardiovascular disease mortality by EMIC tertiles at up to three years of follow-up among individuals aged less than 65 years with ACS in the ERICO cohort, 2009-2013.**

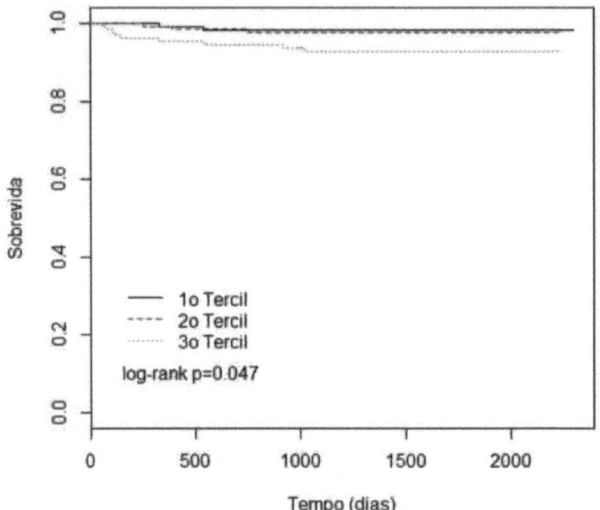

Mean survival time (95% CI) according to the cardiovascular mortality tertiles of the EMIC in individuals under 65 years of age

Tercis IMT (< 65 years)	Events/Individuals	Censored cases	Media (time)		
			Average (days)	95% CI	
				Lower limit	Upper limit
1° (0.40-0.60 mm)	122/2	120 (98.4%)	2.271	2.228	2.315
2° (0.61-0.80 mm)	143/3	140 (97.9%)	2.206	2.160	2.252
3° (0.81-1.50 mm)	135/9	126 (93.3%)	2.095	2.012	2.178

Total	400/14	386 (96.5%)	2.232	2.195	2.268

In the analysis stratified by age, in the group aged <65 years, for mortality from CAD, we found no differences between the survival curves by tertiles of EMIC (*LogRank* = 0.097), as shown in figure 8.

Figure 8 Kaplan-Meier survival curve for mortality from coronary artery disease by the tertiles of the EMIC at up to three years of follow-up among individuals aged less than 65 years with ACS in the ERICO cohort, 2009-2013.

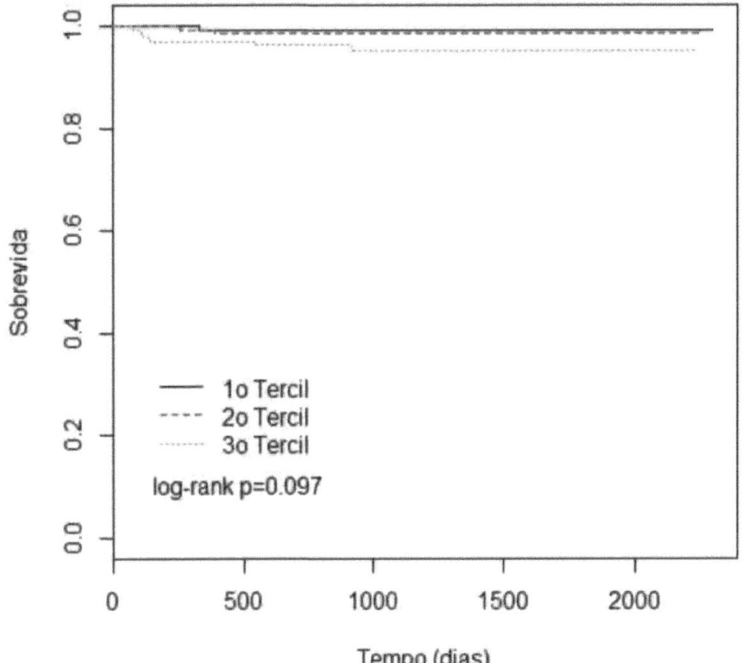

Mean survival time (95% CI) according to mortality from coronary artery disease by tertiles of the EMIC in individuals under 65 years of age

Tercis IMT (< 65 years)	Events/Individuals	Censored cases	Media (time)		
			Average (days)	95% CI	
				Lower limit	Upper limit
1° (0.40-0.60 mm)	122/1	121 (99.2%)	2.286	2.254	2.319

2º (0.61-0.80 mm)	143/2	141 (98.6%)	2.219	2.181	2.257
3° (0.81-1.50 mm)	135/6	129 (95.6%)	2.137	2.066	2.207
Total	400/9	391 (97.8%)	2.256	2.226	2.286

In the analysis stratified by age, in the group aged >65 years, no difference was found between the survival curves by tertiles of EMIC for all-cause mortality, CVD and coronary heart disease, as shown in figures 9-11.

Figure 9. Kaplan-Meier survival curve for all-cause mortality by EMIC tertiles at up to three years of follow-up among individuals aged 65 and over with ACS in the ERICO cohort, 2009-2013.

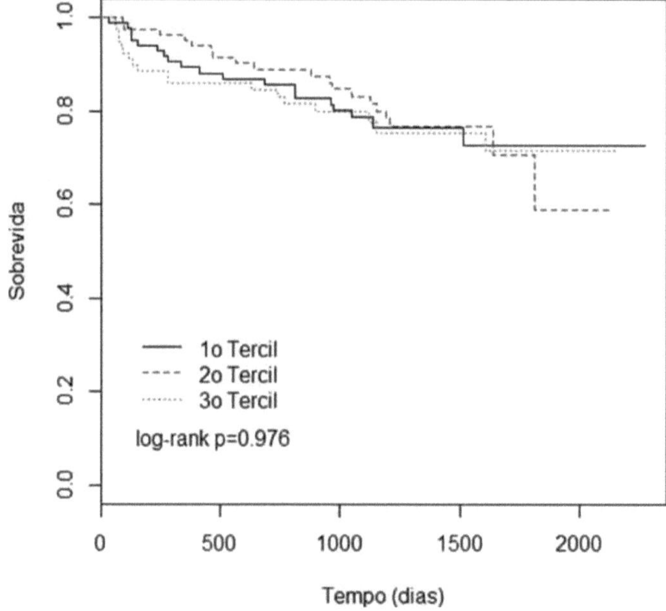

Mean survival time (95% CI) according to all-cause mortality by EMIC tertiles in individuals aged 65 and over				
			Media (time)	
Tercis IMT (> 65 years)	Events/Individuals	Censored cases	Average (days)	95% CI

				Lower limit	Upper limit
1° (0.50-0.80 mm)	84/19	65 (77.4%)	1.842	1.669	2.015
2° (0.81-0.90 mm)	82/20	62 (75.6%)	1.736	1.586	1.887
3° (0.91-1.90 mm)	78/18	60 (76.9%)	1.727	1.549	1.905
Total	244/57	187 (76.6%)	1.825	1.721	1.928

Figure 10 Kaplan-Meier survival curve for cardiovascular disease mortality by EMIC tertiles at up to three years of follow-up among individuals aged 65 years and over with ACS in the ERICO cohort, 2009-2013.

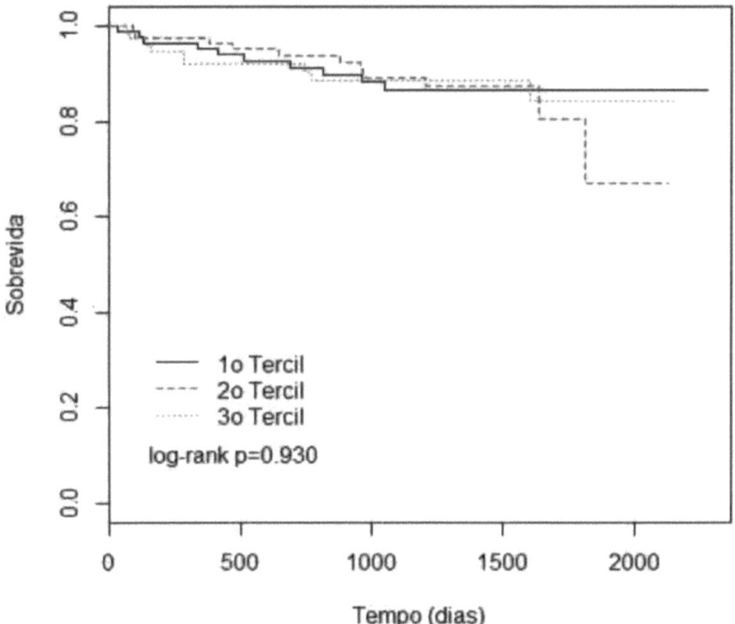

Mean survival time (95% CI) according to cardiovascular mortality by EMIC tertiles in individuals aged 65 and over						
				Media (time)		
Tercis IMT (> 65 years)	Events/Individuals	Censored cases			95% CI	
			Average (days)		Imite inferior	Upper limit
1° (0.50-0.80 mm)	84/10	74 (88.1%)	2.046		1.910	2.181
2° (0.81-0.90 mm)	82/12	70 (85.4%)	1.868		1.730	2.005
3° (0.91-1.90 mm)	78/9	69 (88.5%)	1.933		1.790	2.076
Total	244/31	213 (87.3%)	2.013		1.925	2.101

Figure 11 Kaplan-Meier survival curve for mortality from coronary artery disease by the tertiles of the EMIC at up to three years of follow-up among individuals aged 65 or over affected by ACS in the ERICO cohort, 2009-2013.

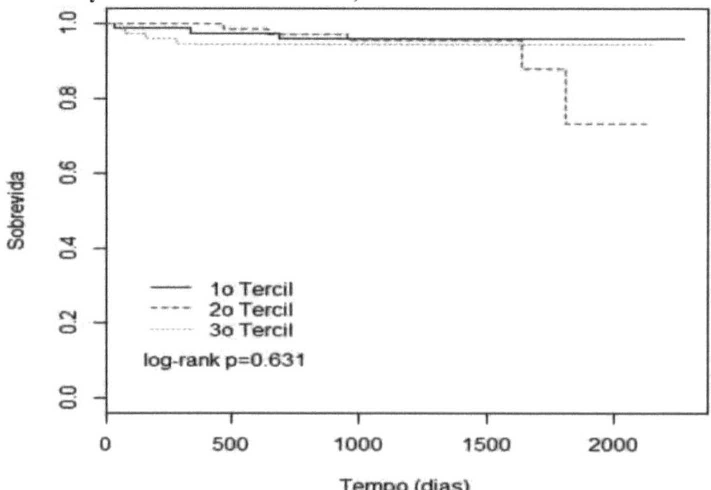

Tercis IMT (> 65 years)	Events /Individuals	Censored cases	Media (time)		
				95%CI	
			Average (days)	Lower limit	Upper limit
1° (0.50-0.80 mm)	84/3	81 (96.4%)	2.204	2.121	2.286
2° (0.81-0.90 mm)	82/6	76 (92.7%)	1.983	1.8692	.097
3° (0.91-1.90 mm)	78/4	74 (94.6%)	2.058	1.954	2.162
Total	244/13	231 (94.7%)	2.153	2.085	2.221

Mean survival time (95% CI) according to coronary artery disease mortality by EMIC tertiles in individuals aged 65 and over.

The analysis stratified by age (<65 years and >65 years) did not represent significance after multivariate adjustment (group <65 years shown in tables 7,8 and 9 - Group >65 years shown in tables 10,11e12).

In an attempt to find some associations, we reproduced the sensitivity analysis excluding cases with EMIC > 1.5, which characterizes atherosclerotic plaque, but after sensitivity analysis our results did not change.

Table 7. Risk Ratio (RR) [95% Confidence Interval (CI)] of all-cause mortality in participants aged <65 years in the ERICO cohort according to EMIC tertiles, 2009-2013.

All causes	1 year Risk ratio 95%CI	2 years Risk ratio 95%CI	3 years Risk ratio 95%CI
No adjustment			
1st tertile	Reference (1,00)	Reference (1,00)	Reference (1,00)
2° tertile	0.86 (0.12-6.13)	0.86 (0.17-4.27)	1.28 (0.36-4.52)
3° tertile	2.81 (0.57-13.91)	2.53 (0.67-9.52)	2.30(0.72-7.32)
Age adjustment			
1st tertile	Reference (1,00)	Reference (1,00)	Reference (1,00)
2° tertile	0.55 (0.76-4.05)	0.58 (0.11-2.95)	1.00 (0.27-3.66)

3° tertile	1.65 (0.32-8.53)	1.56 (0.40-6.14)	1.70 (0.51-5.70)
Adjustment by age and gender			
1st tertile	Reference (1,00)	Reference (1,00)	Reference (1,00)
2° tertile	0.53 (0.07-3.92)	0.57 (0.11-2.91)	1.00 (0.27-3.67)
3° tertile	1.58 (0.30-8.19)	1.53 (0.39-6.03)	1.70 (0.51-5.72)
Multivariate adjustment			
1st tertile	Reference (1,00)	Reference (1,00)	Reference (1,00)
2° tertile	0.26 (0.02-3.12)	0.46 (0.08-2.52)	0.87(0.23-3.34)
3° tertile	1.53 (0.27-8.75)	1.44 (0.34-6.08)	1.63 (0.46-5.81)
1st tertile: 0.40-0.60 mm, 2° tertile: 0.61 -0.80 mm and 3° tertile >0.81 mm.			
Multivariate adjustment: age, gender, education, hypertension, diabetes, dyslipidemia and smoking.			

Table 8. Risk Ratio (RR) [95% Confidence Interval (CI)] of mortality from cardiovascular diseases in participants aged <65 years in the ERICO cohort according to EMIC tertiles, 2009-2013.

Cardiovascular Diseases	1 year Risk ratio 95%CI	2 years Risk ratio 95%CI	3 years Risk ratio 95%CI
No adjustment			
1st tertile	Reference (1,00)	Reference (1,00)	Reference (1,00)
2º tertile	0.87(0.05-13.82)	0.86 (0.12-6.12)	1.28 (0.21-7.68)
3º tertile	5.61 (0.68-46.60)	3.30(0.69-15.91)	4.16(0.90-19.28)
Age adjustment			
1st tertile	Reference (1,00)	Reference (1,00)	Reference (1,00)

2° tertile	0.48 (0.03-7.77)	0.57 (0.08-4.14)	1.00 (0.16-6.17)
3° tertile	2.79 (0.33-23.76)	1.99 (0.40-10.02)	3.04 (0.62-14.90)
Adjustment by age and gender			
1st tertile	Reference (1,00)	Reference (1,00)	Reference (1,00)
2° tertile	0.46 (0.03-7.55)	0.56 (0.08-4.07)	1.00 (0.16-6.20)
3° tertile	2.71 (0.32-23.10)	1.94 (0.39-9.81)	3.06 (0.62-15.01)
Multivariate adjustment			
1st tertile	Reference (1,00)	Reference (1,00)	Reference (1,00)
2° tertile	0.41 (0.02-7.17)	0.42 (0.05-3.38)	0.80 (0.12-5.29)
3° tertile	2.33 (0.25-21.60)	1.67 (0.31-9.14)	2.57 (0.50-13.35)

1st tertile: 0.40-0.60 mm, 2° tertile: 0.61 -0.80 mm and 3° tertile >0.81 mm.

Multivariate adjustment: age, gender, education, hypertension, diabetes, dyslipidemia and smoking.

Table 9. Risk Ratio (RR) [95% Confidence Interval (CI)] of mortality from coronary artery disease in participants aged <65 years in the ERICO cohort according to EMIC tertiles, 2009-2013.

	1 year	2 years	3 years
Coronary Artery Disease	**Risk ratio CI 5th/$_{90}$**	**Risk ratio CI $_{095/o}$**	**Risk ratio CI $_{095/o}$**
No adjustment			
1st tertile	Reference (1,00)	Reference (1,00)	Reference (1,00)
2° tertile	0.87(0.05-13.82)	0.86 (0.05-13.80)	1.72 (0.16-18.95)

3° tertile	3.74 (0.42-33.46)	4.73 (0.55-40.47)	5.59 (0.67-46.44)
Age adjustment			
1st tertile	Reference (1,00)	Reference (1,00)	Reference (1,00)
2° tertile	0.53 (0.03-8.69)	0.52 (0.03-8.57)	1.31 (0.11-15.10)
3° tertile	2.07 (0.22-19.40)	2.60 (0.29-23.18)	4.02 (0.45-35.61)
Adjustment by age and gender			
1st tertile	Reference (1,00)	Reference (1,00)	Reference (1,00)
2° tertile	0.52 (0.03-8.66)	0.51 (0.03-8.43)	1.35 (0.12-15.47)
3° tertile	2.06 (0.22-19.33)	2.55 (0.29-22.76)	4.14(0.47-36.79)

Multivariate adjustment			
1st tertile	Reference (1,00)	Reference (1,00)	Reference (1,00)
2° tertile	0.47 (0.03-8.39)	0.40 (0.02-7.25)	1.05 (0.08-13.36)
3° tertile	1.74 (0.16-18.81)	2.41 (0.25-23.62)	3.66 (0.38-35.76)
1st tertile: 0.40-0.60 mm, 2° tertile: 0.61 -0.80 mm and 3° tertile >0.81 mm.			
Multivariate adjustment: age, gender, education, hypertension, diabetes, dyslipidemia and smoking.			

Table 10. Risk Ratio (RR) [95% Confidence Interval (CI)] of all-cause mortality in participants aged >65 years in the ERICO cohort according to EMIC tertiles, 2009-2013.			
	1 year	2 years	3 years

All cases	Risk ratio CI 5th/$_{90}$	Risk ratio CI 5th/$_{90}$	Risk ratio CI 0$_{95/0}$
No adjustment			
1st tertile	Reference (1,00)	Reference (1,00)	Reference (1,00)
2° tertile	0.45 (0.14-1.45)	0.75 (0.32-1.78)	0.76 (0.37-1.56)
3° tertile	1.37 (0.57-3.32)	1.12(0.50-2.48)	0.99 (0.50-1.98)
Age adjustment 1st tertile	Reference (1,00)	Reference (1,00)	Reference (1,00)
2° tertile	0.44 (0.14-1.44)	0.75 (0.31-1.77)	0.76 (0.37-1.56)
3° tertile	1.30 (0.56-3.13)	1.06 (0.48-2.37)	0.94 (0.47-1.89)
Adjustment by age and gender			

1st tertile	Reference (1,00)	Reference (1,00)	Reference (1,00)
2° tertile	0.45 (0.14-1.46)	0.75 (0.32-1.79)	0.76 (0.37-1.57)
3° tertile	1.30 (0.54-3.16)	1.07 (0.78-2.39)	0.94 (0.47-1.89)
Multivariate adjustment 1st tertile	Reference (1,00)	Reference (1,00)	Reference (1,00)
2° tertile	0.34 (0.09-1.32)	0.70 (0.27-1.78)	0.61 (0.27-1.38)
3° tertile	1.14 (0.43-3.03)	0.88 (0.37-2.13)	0.77 (0.35-1.66)
1st tertile: 0.50-0.80 mm, 2° tertile: 0.81 -0.90 mm and 3° tertile >0.91 mm.			
Multivariate adjustment: age, gender, education, hypertension, diabetes, dyslipidemia and smoking.			

Table 11. Risk Ratio (RR) [Confidence Interval (CI95%)] of cardiovascular disease mortality in participants aged >65 years in the ERICO cohort according to EMIC tertiles, 2009-2013.

Cardiovascular Diseases	1 year Risk ratio 95%CI	2 years Risk ratio 95%CI	3 years Risk ratio 95%CI
No adjustment			
1st tertile	Reference (1,00)	Reference (1,00)	Reference (1,00)
2nd tertile	0.50 (0.09-2.74)	0.71 (0.23-2.25)	0.79 (0.31-2.01)
3rd tertile	1.69 (0.48-5.97)	0.96 (0.32-2.84)	0.90 (0.35-2.28)
Age adjustment			

1st tertile	Reference (1,00)	Reference (1,00)	Reference (1,00)
2nd tertile	0.50 (0.09-2.72)	0.71 (0.23-2.24)	0.79 (0.31-2.00)
3rd tertile	1.57(0.44-5.59)	0.90 (0.30-2.70)	0.84 (0.33-2.14)
Adjustment by age and gender			
1st tertile	Reference (1,00)	Reference (1,00)	Reference (1,00)
2nd tertile	0.53 (0.10-2.88)	0.72 (0.23-2.29)	0.79 (0.31-2.01)
3rd tertile	1.62 (0.45-5.79)	0.91 (0.31-2.73)	0.84 (0.33-2.14)
Multivariate adjustment			

Table 12. Risk Ratio (RR) [95% Confidence Interval (CI)] of mortality from coronary artery disease in participants aged >65 years in the ERICO cohort according to EMIC tertiles, 2009-2013.

Coronary Artery Disease	1 year Risk ratio 95%CI	2 years Risk ratio 95%CI	3 years Risk ratio 95%CI
1st tertile	Reference (1,00)	Reference (1,00)	Reference (1,00)
2nd tertile	0.53 (0.08-3.28)	0.74 (0.22-2.52)	0.76 (0.27-2.08)
3rd tertile	1.45 (0.33-6.48)	0.84 (0.25-2.80)	0.74 (0.26-2.07)

1st tertile: 0.50-0.80 mm, 2nd tertile: 0.81 -0.90 mm and 3rd tertile >0.91 mm.

Multivariate adjustment: age, gender, education, hypertension, diabetes, dyslipidemia and smoking.

No adjustment			
1st tertile	Reference (1,00)	Reference (1,00)	Reference (1,00)
2° tertile	0.00 (0.00-0.00)	0.67 (0.11-3.99)	1.00 (0.20-4.94)
3° tertile	2.21 (0.40-12.06)	1.47 (0.33-6.55)	1.47 (0.33-6.58)
Age adjustment			
1st tertile	Reference (1,00)	Reference (1,00)	Reference (1,00)
2° tertile	0.00 (0.00-0.00)	0.67 (0.11-3.98)	0.99 (0.20-4.89)
3° tertile	2.09 (0.38-11.44)	1.41 (0.31-6.31)	1.37 (0.31-6.15)
Adjustment by age and gender			
1st tertile	Reference (1,00)	Reference (1,00)	Reference (1,00)

2° tertile	0.00 (0.00-0.00)	0.62 (0.10-3.73)	0.90 (0.18-4.48)
3° tertile	1.99 (0.36-10.90)	1.34(0.30-6.00)	1.32 (0.29-5.89)
Multivariate adjustment			
1st tertile	Reference (1,00)	Reference (1,00)	Reference (1,00)
2° tertile	0.00 (0.00-0.00)	1.12(0.15-8.16)	1.12 (0.15-8.16)
3° tertile	3.24 (0.34-31.06)	2.09 (0.37-11.81)	2.09 (0.37-11.81)
1st tertile: 0.50-0.80 mm, 2° tertile: 0.81 -0.90 mm and 3° tertile >0.91 mm.			
Multivariate adjustment: age, gender, education, hypertension, diabetes, dyslipidemia and smoking.			

Chapter 6

6. DISCUSSION

6.1   Main findings

In this study, there was a positive association between traditional cardiovascular risk factors such as hypertension, diabetes and dyslipidemia with the highest tertile of CIMT (>0.81 mm) in the entire sample. In addition, the progressive effect of aging was observed in the CIMT above 0.71 mm (above the 2nd tertile). Low schooling was also associated with higher CIMT. Although we noted almost 61% of men in the tertile of highest CIMT, the association with gender was not significant. Other clinical comorbidities, including smoking and ACS subtypes, were not related to CIMT in this sample. Although our mortality rates in general were associated with high CIMT values, after adjusting mainly for age, this effect was no longer significant. Adjustments for race and ACS subtypes also altered our results.

6.2   EMIC as a predictor of cardiovascular risk

As in our study, previous studies have also described that increased CIMT is associated with ageing (O'Leary et al, 1996; Stein et al, 2008; IBGE, 2010), as well as with traditional CVRF (Andreas et al, 2003; Lorenz et al, 2006). Since atherosclerosis is a systemic disease, carotid atherosclerosis may also reflect the development of this process in coronary arteries and vice versa, and CIMT may be more associated with the severity of ACS than with mortality (Demircan et al, 2005; Ciccone et al, 2013; Rosa et al, 2003). However, we found no association between high CIMT values according to ACS subtypes.

Increases in CIMT were observed in patients with CAD compared to those without previous coronary heart disease. However, differences between the studies that evaluated CIMT, including populations with coronary heart disease, can be explained by the lack of precise definition of the carotid segment studied, the CIMT measurement protocol and the heterogeneity of the studies on age distribution (Lorenz et al, 2007). Probably the lack of standardization of protocols, as some prefer to study the internal carotid artery, others the common carotid artery and some even the carotid bulb, has an influence on the association between CME and CAD.

Given that the conflicting results of standardization are also reflected in the divergent recommendations of some internationally accepted guidelines, for example, the 2010 *American Heart Association / American College of Cardiology* (AHA / ACC) guidelines recommended carotid CME measurements for CVD risk assessment in adults with intermediate risk symptoms (Greenland et al, 2010). The European Society of Hypertension / European Society of Cardiology recommends ultrasound of the carotid arteries to detect vascular hypertrophy or atherosclerosis as a class IIa recommendation with level of evidence B (Mancia et al, 2014). An update of the Mannheim Consensus on Plaques and Carotid Intima-Media Thickness stated that carotid CME measurements and plaque presence are recommended for the initial detection of CVD risk in asymptomatic or intermediate-risk patients (Touboul et al, 2011). However, in 2013, the AHA / ACC guidelines made recommendations against the use of carotid CME for individual risk prediction in clinical practice (Goff et al, 2014).

In our analysis, for example, the CME of all the individuals was carried out in exactly the same place in the common carotid artery (exactly 10 mm anterior to the carotid bulb), regardless of whether there was plaque there or not, which increases the standardization of our analyses. Another difficulty encountered in the development of this study is that, particularly in ACS, few studies have investigated the association with CIMT (Rosa et al, 2003; Demircan et al, 2005; Ciccone et al, 2013), perhaps due to the obviousness of this association, but what caught our attention is that these associations, if proven, could help in the therapy and prognosis of individuals after an ACS event, increasing their survival.

Another obstacle to choosing CIMT for risk prediction is the great influence of age on CIMT, as we found in our own results. In a recent issue of the *Journal of the American Heart Association*, Polak et al (2017) describe an interesting approach to overcoming this problem. They found that a similar approach, creating normative values for EMIC, was well suited to compensate for the generally skewed distribution of EMIC measurements and allowed for the generation of age-specific normative values. Based on data from participants in the Multi-Ethnic Study of Atherosclerosis (MESA), they generated age-, gender- and race-specific normative values for EMIC and were therefore able to compare an individual's measurement as a percentile value, while taking age, gender and ethnic differences into account. The main hypothesis was that an approach using a combined normative percentile score from combined common and internal carotid artery EMI measurements could improve the prediction of CVD events beyond that obtained by a traditional risk factor score, In addition, if the prediction improved independently of the calcium score, the calcium score could be used less, reducing the invasion of patients.

Haberka et al (2017) developed a strategy using EMIC combined with some other factors, mentioned briefly above, in 215 patients, 80 men and
135 women with a mean age of 61.8 ± 7.9 years. Detailed clinical characteristics, including various obesity parameters and the following ultrasound indices were obtained: carotid intima-media thickness (CIMT) and extra-media thickness (EEM), epicardial fat thickness (EGE) and intra-abdominal fat thickness. All these indices were obtained and used in the analysis as separate average values. With them, they developed the *"Periarterial Adipose Tissue Intima Media Adventitia"* (PATIMA) index, which was first described in the study by Haberka and Gasior (2015) and is currently calculated according to the following formula: PATIMA [u] = (EEM/IMC x 35) + EIMC + (EGE x 60). All of the single ultrasound measurements represent different tissue components of the arterial wall and provide different indications of the patient's cardiovascular risk. With this study, Haberka et al (2017) were the first to present a study showing that a combination of ultrasound indices related to periarterial fat and the vascular wall (PATIMA index) is associated with more complex CAD in high and very high risk patients. The PATIMA index showed an improved predictive value compared to other single ultrasound indices and clinical risk assessment.

The population investigated in the MESA, which includes men and women aged between 45 and 84 of varying ethnic origin at six sites in the United States. Of the 6,814 MESA participants, 314 were excluded due to incomplete risk factor or ultrasound examination. In the resulting 6,500 participants, 429 coronary events were recorded during an average follow-up of 10.2 years. They found that the EMIC score significantly improved event prediction.

In the multivariate Cox proportional hazards regression model, the EMIC score combined with age, sex and race proved to be better, increasing the base model statistic from 0.7276 to 0.7457 (P<0.001). Similarly, the logistic regression model had an area under the curve of 0.7210 which increased to 0.7396 (P<0.001) when the combined EMIC score was added to the model. The improvement in prediction achieved by including EMIC was still significant, although slightly attenuated, when the coronary artery calcium index was included in the statistical models.

The take on the problem of CIMT as a risk factor that changes with age presented by Polak et al in the current issue is intriguing (Folsom et al, 2008). This approach significantly increased the prediction of CHD events beyond traditional CVRF, even when the coronary artery calcium score was included in the model. This could potentially revitalize the discussion about CIMT measurements as a viable method for improving CAD prediction. Improving the tools to identify individuals at higher risk is important, especially with regard to CAD, because effective preventive treatment is available. Improving the accuracy of risk prediction can therefore help target those most likely to benefit from preventive treatment. On the other hand, correctly identifying low-risk individuals who do not need primary preventive treatment is of great interest - both for the individual who can be spared preventive treatment and its possible side-effects, and for the community, to ensure that the resources put into healthcare are spent as efficiently as possible. The findings presented by Polak et al are a step towards refining CIMT measurements as an appropriate tool (Folsom et al, 2008) - both by using normative carotid IMT scores and by obtaining greater benefit from a combined common and internal carotid artery CIMT score. As previously mentioned, measuring CIMT is safe, non-invasive and, although it requires some experience, has a fairly high reproducibility.

Furthermore, the normative values calculated from the MESA cohort are not universal, and efforts to generate appropriate normative values in other populations should be encouraged. Further efforts should also include individuals under the age of 45, where the potential for primary prevention may be even greater. And although the improved prediction of CAD obtained by EMIC measurements in this study is promising, these findings need to be replicated for validation.

6.3   EMIC and SCA

Demircan et al. evaluated CIMT in patients with stable angina and patients with ACS subtypes. In this study it was reported that atherosclerotic plaques in the carotid artery and increased CIMT were more frequent in patients who had early onset CAD compared to angina subjects (40% vs 11%, P <0.001, and 0.73 ± 0.10 *vs 0.*60 ± 0.10 mm, P <0.001, respectively). Patients with ACS had significantly increased CIMT compared to patients with stable angina (0.76 ± 0.10 vs 0.70 ± 0.10 mm, P <0.05). The CIMT values reported in this study (Demircan et al, 2005) were similar to those found in our study (mean value of 0.74 mm).

Ciccone et al evaluated CIMT in acute and chronic CAD in a small sample of 133 consecutive patients (mean age 65 ± 9 years). According to the results of this study, higher EMIC values were reported in ACS compared to the chronic CAD group (0.94

± 0.22 vs. 0.86 ± 0.15 mm, P = 0.027) (Ciccone et al, 2013).

Finally, a small national case-control study (Rosa et al, 2003) evaluated EMIC in 29 patients with coronary heart disease (CHD) compared to 29 controls and again found higher EMIC values in CHD cases compared to controls (0.81 +/- 0.25 millimeters and 0.62 +/- 0.18 millimeters, p = 0.001, respectively).

6.4   The prognostic value of EMIC in ACS

With regard to the prognostic value of EMIC and ACS, two previous studies have evaluated mortality (Held et al, 2001; Tello- Montoliu et al, 2007).

The Angina Prognosis Study in Stockholm (APSIS) prospectively evaluated 809 patients with stable angina during double-blind treatment with verapamil or metoprolol. CME, vessel diameter, vessel lumen and plaques in the carotid and femoral arteries were assessed in a subgroup of 558 patients (67% male; mean age: 60 years) in relation to the risk of cardiovascular death (n = 18), non-fatal acute myocardial infarction (n = 26) or myocardial revascularization (n = 70) during three years of follow-up. Similar to our results, Cox regression analysis in the general analysis showed that EMIC, as a continuous variable and plaques, was associated with the risk of death from CVD, as well as non-fatal CAD. However, after adjusting for age, gender, smoking, previous CVD and dyslipidemia, EMIC was a weak predictor of CVD events in individuals with stable angina (p = 0.056) (Held et al, 2001), as were our results after adjustment.

Montoliu et al also studied a small sample of 126 individuals (63.5% male; mean age: 67 years) admitted to the emergency department with non-ST-segment elevation ACS. The carotid artery was assessed using B-mode ultrasound, measuring the EMIC in the posterior wall of the common carotid artery, as in our study. After carrying out these evaluations, they checked the main outcomes (death from CVD, recurrent ACS or revascularization) in six patients.

months of follow-up. In the total sample, 46% had an EMIC equal to or greater than 0.80 and this value was correlated with the TIMI risk score (Pearson r: 0.26; p=0.004). Similar to our

In our results, high EMIC was associated with aging (65 years of age or older) and diabetes; however, no relationship was found between EMIC and mortality in this study (Tello-Montoliu et al, 2007). Regardless of differences in methodology and sample characteristics comparing these previous studies (Held et al, 2001; Tello-Montoliu et al, 2007) with ours, it is suggested that there is no relationship between CIMT and mortality in post-ACS patients. Some hypotheses that may justify these null results, including those presented in our study, may be that CIMT is a better marker of subclinical atherosclerosis in the early stages of coronary disease and is therefore a poor predictor of mortality in this group of patients, even at higher values compared to individuals with more stable CAD (Demircan et al, 2005, Ciccone et al, 2013, Rosa et al, 2003).

6.5   Forces

Although many previous studies have described CVRF-related CIMT and the value of CIMT to predict cardiovascular risk in individuals with intermediate asymptomatic risk (47), the role of CIMT is still not clearly defined in ACS mortality

(Held et al, 2001; Tello-Montoliu et al, 2007). To the best of our knowledge, this is the first study to evaluate the prognostic value of EMIC in an ACS population with low socioeconomic status in Latin America. Previous studies evaluating the prognostic value of EMIC among individuals with ACS have been carried out in developed countries, with different lifestyle habits and CVRF frequencies, as well as socioeconomic status (Held et al, 2001; Tello-Montoliu et al, 2007).

Observational and interventional methods for detecting atherosclerosis of the vessels are widely used in clinical practice, and EMIC measurement is recommended by the AHA as the easiest and most useful method for identifying atherosclerosis due to several factors mentioned above (Smith et al, 2000). EMIC can be measured by B-mode ultrasound, which is a non-invasive, simple and low-cost method that can be performed at any time to investigate in real time the EMIC of the entire carotid complex as indicators of atherosclerosis, including in the femoral arteries, which are also easily accessible, just as we did with the common carotid artery.

In our analysis, we followed a strict protocol for measuring the CIMT of all individuals, which were analyzed at exactly the same location (10mm distal - anterior to the carotid bulb - of the posterior wall of the common carotid artery), regardless of whether or not atherosclerotic plaque was present at that location, which increases the standardization of our analyses.

6.6   Limit

Analyses including other cardiovascular outcomes, particularly non-fatal events such as recurrence of a new non-fatal AMI, coronary artery bypass grafting or percutaneous transluminal coronary angioplasty (PTCA), were not considered in this analysis.

Although the definition of a carotid segment improves the standardization of the assessment, some of the high EMIC values may be due to the presence of plaque. However, when we excluded EMIC values >1.5 mm, our findings did not change. In fact, the inclusion in the 3rd tertile of individuals with probable established plaque could have favored a positive association between EMIC and worse survival after ACS. Therefore, our null result suggests that it is true.

Another limitation of this study is that we did not include other measures, such as the analysis of carotid plaques, which could have greater predictive power in terms of mortality in patients with ACS. In fact, there is a scarcity of publications evaluating the prognostic value of carotid CME and mortality after ACS (Held et al, 2001; Tello- Montoliu et al, 2007).

Although CIMT is the most commonly used surrogate marker for atherosclerosis in the general population without previous CAD, the presence of carotid plaque added to the CIMT assessment may be useful for risk stratification in CAD patients in the field of secondary prevention, including ACS.

Prospective data from the ERICO cohort should add valuable information on CME and carotid plaques and their prognostic value with other cardiovascular outcomes, such as recurrence of a non-fatal AMI, coronary artery bypass grafting or angioplasty.

CONCLUSION

The results of this study show that EMIC was mainly associated with aging. As expected, traditional cardiovascular risk factors such as hypertension, diabetes and dyslipidemia were also more frequent among post-ACS participants with the highest EMIC values (3° tertile), regardless of the ACS subtype. However, EMIC did not prove to be a good weak predictor of all-cause mortality, CVD and CAD in the short and long term.

PERSPECTIVES

To analyze plaques in the common carotid artery and bulb in the ultrasound scans of the individuals participating in the ERICO study in order to verify whether the presence of carotid plaque would have a greater association with mortality in post-ACS individuals.

ANNEXES

Annex 1

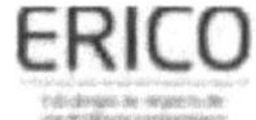

Hospital Universitário | Centro de Pesquisa Clínica
Av. Lineu Prestes 2565 / 2° andar | Cidade Universitária
Butantã, São Paulo, Brasil 05508-000
Fone: 55-11 3091-9300 | Fax: 55-11 3091-9241

PROJETO INSUFICIÊNCIA CORONARIANA

Termo de Consentimento Livre e Esclarecido (TCLE)

Apresentação do estudo:

O Projeto ERICO (Estratégia de Registro da Insuficiência Coronariana) é uma pesquisa sobre a doença coronariana que acomete a população adulta, como o infarto (ataque do coração). É um estudo que será realizado no Hospital Universitário – USP e acompanhará os casos de infarto que chegarem ao hospital para avaliação das condições de saúde nos pacientes com essa coronariana.

Participação no estudo:

O/A Sr./a é convidado/a a participar do estudo que envolve o acompanhamento dos participantes por pelo menos dois anos, com a realização de entrevistas por telefone ou presencial no Hospital Universitário-USP ao final do primeiro mês depois do infarto, dos primeiros 6 meses e depois anualmente.

Inicialmente, o/a Sr./a fará a primeira parte da entrevista logo após a chegada ao hospital. Enquanto o Sr(a) estiver internado será coletado sangue para realização de exames. Junto com a realização desses exames serão colhidos mais 30 ml de sangue, 10 ml de saliva, 10 ml de urina que ficarão guardados para exames a serem realizados no futuro, incluindo extração de DNA e RNA, em ocasiões distintas (durante internação e pós 30 dias do infarto). O total de sangue coletado não traz inconveniências para adultos. Apenas um leve desconforto pode ocorrer associado à picada da agulha. Algumas vezes pode haver sensação momentânea de tontura ou pequena reação local, mas esses efeitos são passageiros e não oferecem riscos. Esse sangue guardado é fundamental para futuras análises que possam ampliar o conhecimento sobre as doenças em estudo.

Após esta primeira etapa do estudo, o/a Sr./a. será periodicamente contatado/a por telefone, correspondência ou e-mail para acompanhar as modificações no seu estado de saúde e para obtenção de informações adicionais. Por isso, é muito importante informar seu novo endereço e telefone em caso de mudança. Para poder monitorar melhor sua situação de saúde, é essencial ter acesso ao seu prontuário médico caso o Sr(a) apresente algum problema de saúde depois da alta.

Análises adicionais, de caráter genético ou não, que não foram incluídas nos objetivos definidos no protocolo original da pesquisa, somente serão realizadas mediante a apresentação de projetos de pesquisa específicos, aprovados pelo Comitê de Ética da instituição incluindo a assinatura de novos Termos de Consentimento Livre e Esclarecido.

Seus direitos como participante:

Sua participação é inteiramente voluntária. Todos os procedimentos realizados serão inteiramente gratuitos. Todos os resultados dos exames realizados serão entregues ao Sr(a).

Todas as informações obtidas do/a Sr/a. serão confidenciais, identificadas por um número e sem menção ao seu nome. Elas serão utilizadas exclusivamente para fins de análise científica e serão guardadas com segurança - somente terão acesso a elas os pesquisadores envolvidos no projeto.

Uma cópia deste Termo de Consentimento lhe será entregue. Se houver perguntas ou necessidade de mais informações sobre o estudo, ou qualquer intercorrência, o/a Sr/a. pode procurar o Professor Paulo Andrade Lotufo, Professora Isabela Benseñor ou Dra Alessandra Carvalho Goulart no Hospital Universitário – USP na Av. Lineu Prestes 2565, telefone (11) 3091-9271 coordenadores do projeto no CI-SP. O Comitê de Ética e Pesquisa do Hospital Universitário da USP pode ser contatado pelo seguinte telefone: (11) 3091-9457.

Sua assinatura abaixo significa que o/a Sr/a. leu e compreendeu todas as informações e concorda em participar da pesquisa.

Termo de Consentimento Livre e Esclarecido

Nome do/a participante: ....

Documento de Identidade: ....

Data de nascimento: ....

Endereço: ....

Telefones para contato:...

Declaro que compreendi as informações apresentadas neste documento e dei meu consentimento para participação no estudo.

Autorizo os pesquisadores do estudo a obter informações sobre a ocorrência de hospitalizações, licenças médicas, eventos de saúde, aposentadoria, ou afastamento de qualquer natureza em registros de saúde junto ao Hospital Universitário - USP e a outras instituições de saúde públicas ou privadas, conforme indicar a situação específica.

No caso de hospitalização, autorizo, adicionalmente, que o/a representante do estudo devidamente credenciado/a, copie dados constantes na papeleta de internação, bem como resultados de exames realizados durante minha internação.

As informações obtidas somente poderão ser utilizadas para fins estatísticos e deverão ser mantidas sob proteção, codificadas e sem minha identificação nominal.

Assinatura____

Local____________________________ Data _______/_______/_______

Nome do/a entrevistador/a: ....

Assinatura: _______________________________

FICHA SEGUIMENTO INICIAL

Nome:_______________________________

Registro ERICO:___________ Data questionário:___________

Entrevistadora:_______________________________

ERICO

NOME	ID ERICO
_______________________________	

DATA DE NASC _______________	SEXO ○ Masculino ○ Feminino	RG HU

Unidade de Ocorrência ○ PA ○ UTI/SEMI ○ Enfermaria	Data de Entrada PS-HU ___________ Hora de Entrada PS-HU ___________	Procedência ○ CASA ○ SAMU ○ UBS	Data ___________ Hora ___________

Cor ou raça? ○ Branco ○ Mulato ou Pardo ○ Negro ○ Asiático	Estado civil ○ Solteiro ○ Casado ○ Divorciado/Separado ○ Viúvo ○ Amigado ○ Ignorado/Não consta	Nível de escolaridade ○ Sem estudo formal ○ Fundamental incompleto ○ Fundamental completo ○ Médio incompleto ○ Médio completo ○ Superior incompleto ○ Superior completo ○ Pós graduação

ANTECEDENTES DE RISCO:

TABAGISMO ○ Tabagista atual ○ Ex-Tabagista ○ Nunca fumou ○ Não sabe ○ DI (dados insuficientes)	Se tabagista atual, quantos cigarros por dia? ________ Se ex-tabagista, por ________	Fuma há quantos anos? ________ Há quanto tempo parou? ________

Uso de cocaína ou crack? ○ Sim ○ Não ○ Não sabe ○ DI	HAS ○ Sim ○ Não ○ Não sabe ○ DI	DM ○ Sim ○ Não ○ Não sabe ○ DI	DISLIPIDEMIA ○ Sim ○ Não ○ Não sabe ○ DI	SEDENTARISMO ○ Sim ○ Não ○ Não sabe ○ DI

INSUFICIÊNCIA RENAL ○ Sim ○ Não ○ Não sabe ○ DI	MENOPAUSA ○ Sim ○ Não ○ Não sabe ○ DI ○ Não se aplica	MENOPAUSA HÁ QUANTOS ANOS	OUTROS ANTECEDENTES?

ICO PREVIA ○ Sim ○ Não ○ Não sabe ○ Sem inf	TIPO DE ICO PREVIA ☐ IAM Previo ☐ ATC Previa ☐ RM Previa ☐ Outros →	SE OUTROS QUAL?	1° EVENTO HÁ QUANTOS ANOS ? IAM Previo [ ] ATC Previa [ ] RM Previa [ ]	CONTRACEPÇÃO OU TRH? ○ Sim ○ Não ○ Não sabe	SE SIM, HÁ QUANTOS ANOS ?

ANTECEDENTE FAMILIAR DE ICO PRECOCE ☐ FAMILIAR MASCULINO < 55 ANOS ☐ FAMILIAR FEMININO < 65 ANOS ☐ NÃO ☐ NÃO SABE ☐ DI	ICC ○ Sim ○ Não ○ Não sabe ○ DI	AVC ○ Sim ○ Não ○ Não sabe ○ DI	APRESENTOU 2 OU MAIS EPISÓDIOS DE DOR PRECORDIAL NAS ÚLTIMAS 24H? ○ Sim ○ Não ○ Não sabe ○ DI

<table>
<tr><td>

Consome café?

○ Sim, com cafeína   ○ Sim, sem cafeína

○ Não   ○ DI

</td><td>

Quantidade consumida por vez (xícaras)?

____

</td></tr>
<tr><td>

Frequência com que consome café?

○ Mais de 3 vezes ao dia

○ 2 a 3 vezes ao dia

○ 1 vez ao dia

○ 5 a 6 vezes na semana

○ 2 a 4 vezes na semana

○ 1 vez na semana

○ 1 a 3 vezes ao mês

○ Nunca/quase nunca

</td><td>

Qual o tipo de café que o senhor usualmente consome?

○ Passado em filtro ou coador

○ Expresso

○ Cafeteira italiana

○ Solúvel (instantâneo)

○ Dados insuficientes

○ Outro, especifique

____

</td></tr>
</table>

ELETROCARDIOGRAMA

DATA DO ECG (DD MM AAAA)		HORA DO ECG (HH MM)	
AINDA COM DOR NO ECG ○ SIM ○ NÃO ○ DI		RITMO SINUSAL? ○ SIM ○ NÃO	

SE NÃO, QUAL RITMO? ______________________________

ALTERAÇÕES DE ST-T

☐ SUPRA   ☐ INFRA   ☐ BRE   ☐ INVERSÃO DE ONDA T   ☐ ECG NORMAL

INFRA ST > 0.05 MM ○ SIM ○ NÃO	ALTERAÇÃO COM NITRATO ○ SIM ○ NÃO ○ Não se aplica	SUPRA > 1MM 2 DERIVAÇÕES ○ SIM ○ NÃO

PAREDE(S) SEGMENTO ST

☐ SEPTAL (V1-V2)   ☐ ANTERIOR (V3-V4)   ☐ LATERAL (V5, V6)   ☐ VD (V3R, V4R)

☐ INFERIOR (II III, AVF)   ☐ DORSAL (V7,V8)   ☐ LAT ALTA (I,AVL)   ☐ ALT DINÂMICA

ONDA Q? ○ SIM ○ NÃO	AMPLITUDE DO MAIOR SUPRA ______________________________ OU INFRA NO ECG ______________________________

PAREDE(S) ONDA Q

☐ SEPTAL (V1-V2)   ☐ ANTERIOR (V3-V4)   ☐ LATERAL (V5, V6)   ☐ VD (V3R, V4R)

☐ INFERIOR (II III, AVF)   ☐ DORSAL (V7,V8)   ☐ LAT ALTA (I,AVL)   ☐ ALT DINÂMICA

OUTRAS ALTERAÇÕES NO ELETRO? ______________________________

DADOS LABORATORIAIS DE ENTRADA

VALORES DE ENTRADA		TROPONINA	
UREIA		1º VALOR	
CREATININA		HORA (1º)	
POTASSIO		MAIOR	
HB		HORA(>)	
HT		CKMB	
LEUCOCITOS		1º VALOR	
EOSINOFILOS(%)		HORA(1º)	
PLAQUETAS		MAIOR	
GLICEMIA		HORA(>)	
HDL		CT	
LDL		TG	

MEDICAÇÃO

MEDICAÇÕES PRÉVIAS (CASA)

☐ AAS ☐ WARFARINA
☐ CLOPIDOGREL ☐ ESTATINA/HIPOLIPEMIANTE
☐ BETA-BLOQUEADOR ☐ FIBRATO
☐ BLOQUEADOR CALCIO ☐ NITRATO
☐ IECA ☐ HIPOGLICEMIANTE ORAL
☐ BRA ☐ INSULINA
☐ DIURETICO ☐ BLOQ BOMBA
☐ ALDACTONE ☐ BLOQ H2

OUTRAS MEDICAÇÕES ?
O SIM O NÃO

QUAL(IS)?

HISTÓRIA QUADRO ATUAL:

EQUIVALENTE ISQUÊMICO		CARACTERÍSTICA DA DOR ATUAL		
O SIM	O NÃO	O TÍPICA	O SUGESTIVA	O ATÍPICA

AINDA COM DOR NA ENTRADA	HORA DE INÍCIO DA DOR	DATA DE INÍCIO DA DOR
O SIM O NÃO		

EXAME FÍSICO DE ENTRADA

DADOS VITAIS:		SATURAÇÃO DE O2 (mm)
PRESSÃO SISTÓLICA (MMHG)	☐	
PRESSÃO DIASTÓLICA (MMHG)	☐	
		KILLIP
FC (BPM)	☐	○ I
ALTURA (CM)	☐	○ II
		○ III
PESO (KG)	☐	○ IV

DIAGNÓSTICO INICIAL (DE ENTRADA)

○ IAM CSST   ○ AI RISCO MÉDIO
○ IAM SSST   ○ AI ALTO RISCO
○ AI BAIXO RISCO   ○ DOR NÃO CORONARIANA

DIAGNÓSTICO DE SAÍDA

IAM sem supra	IAM com supra	Angina instável	Risco AI:	OUTROS. QUAL?
○ Sim ○ Não	○ Sim ○ Não	○ Sim ○ Não	○ Baixo ○ Médio ○ Alto	

ERICO

Hospital Universitário | Centro de Pesquisa Clínica
Av. Lineu Prestes 2565 | 1º andar | Cidade Universitária
Butantã São Paulo Brasil 05508-000
Fone: 55 11 3091 9300 | Fax: 55 11 3091 9290

NOME:____

REGISTRO ERICO:________________

DATA QUESTIONÁRIO:__________________

ENTREVISTADOR: ____

Patient Health Questionnaire: PHQ-9- 30 dias				
Nas últimas duas semanas com que freqüência você se sentiu incomodado por algum dos problemas abaixo?	Nunca (0)	Várias Vezes (1)	Mais da metade dos dias (2)	Quase todo dia (3)
1. Pouco interesse ou prazer em fazer as atividades do dia a dia				
2. Sentindo-se para baixo, deprimido ou sem esperança				
3. problemas para pegar no sono, continuar dormindo ou por dormir demais				
4. Sentindo-se cansado ou com pouca energia				
5. Com pouco apetite ou comendo demais				
6. Sentido mal com você mesmo ou que você é um fracasso ou que você pôs você mesmo ou sua família para baixo				
7. Problemas de concentração, como para ler jornal ou assistir televisão				
8. Está se movimentando ou falando tão devagar que outras pessoas notaram? Ou ao contrário que você está tão agitado ou inquieto que você acaba se movimentando mais do que o habitual				
9. Pensamentos que seria melhor você morrer ou se ferir de alguma maneira				
Escore total =				

Se você apresentou algum problema, o quanto esses problemas atrapalharam você no trabalho, a cuidar das coisas em casa ou na sua relação com outras pessoas

( ) Não atrapalhou
( ) Atrapalhou um pouco
( ) Atrapalhou muito
( ) Atrapalhou demais

Gravidade da depressão de acordo com PHQ-9 escore (preenchimento médico):

Mínima (0 - 4)___________
Leve (5 - 9)___________
Moderada (10 - 14)___________
Moderadamente grave (15 - 19)________
Grave (20 - 27)______________

QUESTIONÁRIO DE FREQUÊNCIA ALIMENTAR (QFA)-30 DIAS

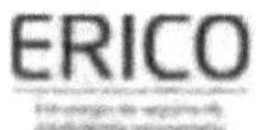

NOME:____REGISTRO ERICO:_______________

DATA QUESTIONÁRIO:_________________

ENTREVISTADOR:____________________________________

QUESTIONÁRIO DE FREQUÊNCIA ALIMENTAR

Nº do Quest

Gostaríamos que você respondesse com que frequência tem comido alguns alimentos, agora que está grávida, e também a quantidade de alimento que come a cada vez.

Primeira pergunta: Com que frequência você tem comido "nome do alimento"?
Caso ela refira consumir o alimento, perguntar: Quantas "ler á medida caseira"?
A cada 4 ou 5 alimentos lembrar a gestante que o questionário se refere alimentação durante a gestação.

Alimento	Quantidade consumida por vez	Mais de 3x/dia	2 a 3 x/dia	1 x/dia	5 a 6 x/sem	2 a 4 x/sem	1 x/sem	1 a 3 x/mês	Nunca/ Quase nunca
Arroz Branco	col sopa ch	3 ☐	2 ☐	1 ☐	0.76 ☐	0.43 ☐	0.14 ☐	0.07 ☐	0 ☐
Arroz Integral	col sopa ch	3 ☐	2 ☐	1 ☐	0.76 ☐	0.43 ☐	0.14 ☐	0.07 ☐	0 ☐
Feijão	concha méd	3 ☐	2 ☐	1 ☐	0.76 ☐	0.43 ☐	0.14 ☐	0.07 ☐	0 ☐
Macarrão	Escumadeira cheia / pegador	3 ☐	2 ☐	1 ☐	0.76 ☐	0.43 ☐	0.14 ☐	0.07 ☐	0 ☐
Macarrão integral	Escumadeira cheia / pequena	3 ☐	2 ☐	1 ☐	0.76 ☐	0.43 ☐	0.14 ☐	0.07 ☐	0 ☐
Farinha de Mandioca	colher sope	3 ☐	2 ☐	1 ☐	0.76 ☐	0.43 ☐	0.14 ☐	0.07 ☐	0 ☐
Pão carioquinha/ frances	frances / 2 fatias pão for	3 ☐	2 ☐	1 ☐	0.76 ☐	0.43 ☐	0.14 ☐	0.07 ☐	0 ☐
Pão integral / centeio	fatia	3 ☐	2 ☐	1 ☐	0.76 ☐	0.43 ☐	0.14 ☐	0.07 ☐	0 ☐
Pão caseiro	fatia	3 ☐	2 ☐	1 ☐	0.76 ☐	0.43 ☐	0.14 ☐	0.07 ☐	0 ☐
Biscoito doce	unidade	3 ☐	2 ☐	1 ☐	0.76 ☐	0.43 ☐	0.14 ☐	0.07 ☐	0 ☐
Bolos-cucas	fatias	3 ☐	2 ☐	1 ☐	0.76 ☐	0.43 ☐	0.14 ☐	0.07 ☐	0 ☐
Biscoito Salgado	unidade	3 ☐	2 ☐	1 ☐	0.76 ☐	0.43 ☐	0.14 ☐	0.07 ☐	0 ☐
Polenta	pedaço	3 ☐	2 ☐	1 ☐	0.76 ☐	0.43 ☐	0.14 ☐	0.07 ☐	0 ☐
Batata Frita ou chips	porção peq	3 ☐	2 ☐	1 ☐	0.76 ☐	0.43 ☐	0.14 ☐	0.07 ☐	0 ☐
Batata cozida	unidade	3 ☐	2 ☐	1 ☐	0.76 ☐	0.43 ☐	0.14 ☐	0.07 ☐	0 ☐
Mandioca aipim	pedaço	3 ☐	2 ☐	1 ☐	0.76 ☐	0.43 ☐	0.14 ☐	0.07 ☐	0 ☐
Milho verde	1 espiga / 4 col sopa	3 ☐	2 ☐	1 ☐	0.76 ☐	0.43 ☐	0.14 ☐	0.07 ☐	0 ☐
Pipoca	xícara	3 ☐	2 ☐	1 ☐	0.76 ☐	0.43 ☐	0.14 ☐	0.07 ☐	0 ☐
Lentilha/ Ervilha/Grão de Bico	colher sopa	3 ☐	2 ☐	1 ☐	0.76 ☐	0.43 ☐	0.14 ☐	0.07 ☐	0 ☐
Alface	folha	3 ☐	2 ☐	1 ☐	0.76 ☐	0.43 ☐	0.14 ☐	0.07 ☐	0 ☐
Couve	col sopa ch	3 ☐	2 ☐	1 ☐	0.76 ☐	0.43 ☐	0.14 ☐	0.07 ☐	0 ☐
Repolho	col sopa ch	3 ☐	2 ☐	1 ☐	0.76 ☐	0.43 ☐	0.14 ☐	0.07 ☐	0 ☐
Laranja/ Bergamota	unidade	3 ☐	2 ☐	1 ☐	0.76 ☐	0.43 ☐	0.14 ☐	0.07 ☐	0 ☐
Banana	unidade	3 ☐	2 ☐	1 ☐	0.76 ☐	0.43 ☐	0.14 ☐	0.07 ☐	0 ☐

Alimento	Quantidade consumida por vez	Mais de 3x/dia	2 a 3 x/dia	1 x/dia	5 a 6 x/sem	2 a 4 x/sem	1 x/sem	1 a 3 x/mês	Nunca/ Quase nunca
Mamão/Papaia	fati 1/2 papaia	3	2	1	0,79	0,43	0,14	0,07	0
Maçã	unidade	3	2	1	0,79	0,43	0,14	0,07	0
Melancia/ Melão	fatia	3	2	1	0,79	0,43	0,14	0,07	0
Abacaxi	fatia	3	2	1	0,79	0,43	0,14	0,07	0
Abacate	1/2 unidade	3	2	1	0,79	0,43	0,14	0,07	0
Manga	unidade	3	2	1	0,79	0,43	0,14	0,07	0
Limão	Só a frequência	3	2	1	0,79	0,43	0,14	0,07	0
Maracujá	Só a frequência	3	2	1	0,79	0,43	0,14	0,07	0
Uva	cacho médio	3	2	1	0,79	0,43	0,14	0,07	0
Goiaba	unidade	3	2	1	0,79	0,43	0,14	0,07	0
Pêra	unidade	3	2	1	0,79	0,43	0,14	0,07	0
Chicórea	col sopa ch	3	2	1	0,79	0,43	0,14	0,07	0
Tomate	unidade	3	2	1	0,79	0,43	0,14	0,07	0
Chuchu	col sopa ch	3	2	1	0,79	0,43	0,14	0,07	0
Abóbora	col sopa ch	3	2	1	0,79	0,43	0,14	0,07	0
Abobrinha	col sopa ch	3	2	1	0,79	0,43	0,14	0,07	0
Pepino	fatia	3	2	1	0,79	0,43	0,14	0,07	0
Vagem	col sopa ch	3	2	1	0,79	0,43	0,14	0,07	0
Cebola	Só a frequência	3	2	1	0,79	0,43	0,14	0,07	0
Alho	Só a frequência	3	2	1	0,79	0,43	0,14	0,07	0
Pimentão	Só a frequência	3	2	1	0,79	0,43	0,14	0,07	0
Cenoura	col sopa ch	3	2	1	0,79	0,43	0,14	0,07	0
Beterraba	fatia	3	2	1	0,79	0,43	0,14	0,07	0
Couve Flor	ramo ou flor	3	2	1	0,79	0,43	0,14	0,07	0
Ovos	unidades	3	2	1	0,79	0,43	0,14	0,07	0
Leite Integral	copo	3	2	1	0,79	0,43	0,14	0,07	0
Leite Semidesnatado	copo	3	2	1	0,79	0,43	0,14	0,07	0
Leite Desnatado	copo	3	2	1	0,79	0,43	0,14	0,07	0
Iogurte Normal	unidade	3	2	1	0,79	0,43	0,14	0,07	0
Iogurte Light	unidade	3	2	1	0,79	0,43	0,14	0,07	0
Queijo	fatia media	3	2	1	0,79	0,43	0,14	0,07	0
Requeijão	Só a frequência	3	2	1	0,79	0,43	0,14	0,07	0
Manteiga	Só a frequência	3	2	1	0,79	0,43	0,14	0,07	0
Margarina	Só a frequência	3	2	1	0,79	0,43	0,14	0,07	0
Vísceras: figado,coração bucho	pedaço	3	2	1	0,79	0,43	0,14	0,07	0

Alimento	Quantidade consumida por vez	Mais de 3x/dia	2 a 3 x/dia	1 x/dia	5 a 6 x/sem	2 a 4 x/sem	1 x/sem	1 a 3 x/mês	Nunca/ Quase nunca
Carne de boi s/osso	☐ , ☐ 1 bife médio = 4 col sopa moída ou 2 pedaços	3 ☐	2 ☐	1 ☐	0,79 ☐	0,43 ☐	0,14 ☐	0,07 ☐	0 ☐
Carne de boi c/osso/mocotó/ rabo	☐ , ☐ pedaço	3 ☐	2 ☐	1 ☐	0,79 ☐	0,43 ☐	0,14 ☐	0,07 ☐	0 ☐
Carne porco	☐ , ☐ pedaço	3 ☐	2 ☐	1 ☐	0,79 ☐	0,43 ☐	0,14 ☐	0,07 ☐	0 ☐
Frango	☐ , ☐ pedaço	3 ☐	2 ☐	1 ☐	0,79 ☐	0,43 ☐	0,14 ☐	0,07 ☐	0 ☐
Salsicha/ lingüiça	☐ , ☐ unid ou gomo	3 ☐	2 ☐	1 ☐	0,79 ☐	0,43 ☐	0,14 ☐	0,07 ☐	0 ☐
Peixe fresco	☐ , ☐ file ou posta	3 ☐	2 ☐	1 ☐	0,79 ☐	0,43 ☐	0,14 ☐	0,07 ☐	0 ☐
Peixe enlatado (atum,sardinha)	☐ , ☐ latas	3 ☐	2 ☐	1 ☐	0,79 ☐	0,43 ☐	0,14 ☐	0,07 ☐	0 ☐
Hambúrguer	☐ , ☐ unidades	3 ☐	2 ☐	1 ☐	0,79 ☐	0,43 ☐	0,14 ☐	0,07 ☐	0 ☐
Pizza	☐ , ☐ pedaço	3 ☐	2 ☐	1 ☐	0,79 ☐	0,43 ☐	0,14 ☐	0,07 ☐	0 ☐
Camarão	☐ , ☐ unidades	3 ☐	2 ☐	1 ☐	0,79 ☐	0,43 ☐	0,14 ☐	0,07 ☐	0 ☐
Bacon/toucinho	☐ , ☐ fatia	3 ☐	2 ☐	1 ☐	0,79 ☐	0,43 ☐	0,14 ☐	0,07 ☐	0 ☐
Maionese	☐ , ☐ colher chá	3 ☐	2 ☐	1 ☐	0,79 ☐	0,43 ☐	0,14 ☐	0,07 ☐	0 ☐
salgados: Kibe,pastel	☐ , ☐ unidades	3 ☐	2 ☐	1 ☐	0,79 ☐	0,43 ☐	0,14 ☐	0,07 ☐	0 ☐
Salgadinhos	☐ , ☐ pacote	3 ☐	2 ☐	1 ☐	0,79 ☐	0,43 ☐	0,14 ☐	0,07 ☐	0 ☐
Sorvete	☐ , ☐ unidades	3 ☐	2 ☐	1 ☐	0,79 ☐	0,43 ☐	0,14 ☐	0,07 ☐	0 ☐
Açúcar	☐ , ☐ col/sobremesa	3 ☐	2 ☐	1 ☐	0,79 ☐	0,43 ☐	0,14 ☐	0,07 ☐	0 ☐
Caramelo, bala	Só a freqüência	3 ☐	2 ☐	1 ☐	0,79 ☐	0,43 ☐	0,14 ☐	0,07 ☐	0 ☐
Chocolate pó/ Nescau	☐ , ☐ col/sobremesa	3 ☐	2 ☐	1 ☐	0,79 ☐	0,43 ☐	0,14 ☐	0,07 ☐	0 ☐
Chocolatebarra/ bombom	☐ , ☐ 1 peq. ou 2 bombons	3 ☐	2 ☐	1 ☐	0,79 ☐	0,43 ☐	0,14 ☐	0,07 ☐	0 ☐
Pudim	☐ , ☐ pedaço	3 ☐	2 ☐	1 ☐	0,79 ☐	0,43 ☐	0,14 ☐	0,07 ☐	0 ☐
Doce de leite/ Geléia	☐ , ☐ col/sobremesa	3 ☐	2 ☐	1 ☐	0,79 ☐	0,43 ☐	0,14 ☐	0,07 ☐	0 ☐
Refrigerante Normal	☐ , ☐ copo	3 ☐	2 ☐	1 ☐	0,79 ☐	0,43 ☐	0,14 ☐	0,07 ☐	0 ☐
Refrigerante Light	☐ , ☐ copo	3 ☐	2 ☐	1 ☐	0,79 ☐	0,43 ☐	0,14 ☐	0,07 ☐	0 ☐
Cafe	☐ , ☐ xícara	3 ☐	2 ☐	1 ☐	0,79 ☐	0,43 ☐	0,14 ☐	0,07 ☐	0 ☐
Suco Natural	☐ , ☐ copo	3 ☐	2 ☐	1 ☐	0,79 ☐	0,43 ☐	0,14 ☐	0,07 ☐	0 ☐
Suco Artificial	☐ , ☐ copo	3 ☐	2 ☐	1 ☐	0,79 ☐	0,43 ☐	0,14 ☐	0,07 ☐	0 ☐
Vinho	☐ , ☐ copo	3 ☐	2 ☐	1 ☐	0,79 ☐	0,43 ☐	0,14 ☐	0,07 ☐	0 ☐
Cerveja	☐ , ☐ copo	3 ☐	2 ☐	1 ☐	0,79 ☐	0,43 ☐	0,14 ☐	0,07 ☐	0 ☐
Outras Bebidas alcoólicas	☐ , ☐ dose	3 ☐	2 ☐	1 ☐	0,79 ☐	0,43 ☐	0,14 ☐	0,07 ☐	0 ☐

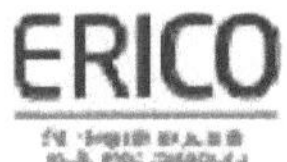

OR COMPLEMENTARY WORKSHOPS

Date of contact:	Interviewer:	
Participant name:		IDERICO:
Segnimento☐ 180 días☐ (llano Oíanos Oíanos☐☐☐ 04 anos		

A J UÄ J. [¿ACÁO 1XJS LATO RES DE RISCO E HÁBITOS DEVIDO

1. Coffee consumption

Al O part ici paute consomé café?

	Yes. rom caffeine		Yes$_r$ without caffeine
	NSo		DI

B} Amount consumed at a time (xfcaras]

C) How often you drink coffee:

	More than 3 times a day		2 to 4 times a week
	2 to 3 times a day		1 time a week
	1 time a day		1 to 3 times a month
	5 to 6 times a week		Never / almost never

D) What kind of coffee do you usually drink?

	Pass through filter or filter		Soluble fmstantaneousD]
	Express yourself		DI
Italian Caíetetra			Or iro íquall:

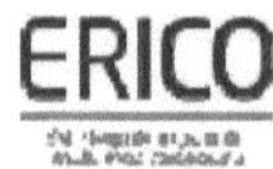

Hospital Universitário | Centro de Pesquisa Clínica
Av. Lineu Prestes 2565 3º andar | Cidade Universitária
Pinheiros, São Paulo, PR 25778-000
Fone: 55 11 2661-6000 | Fax: 55 11 3668-0000

2. Hypertension

Previously available information <u>latest</u>

	Yes
	No
	Doesn't know / DI

Confirmation / data collection <u>in this **segment**</u> ¡mentó

Yes	
No	
You don't know	
DI	
Not applicable (I already had the diagnosis)	

3. Diabetes

Previously available information <u>latest</u>

	Yes
	No
	Doesn't know / DI

Confirmation / data collection <u>in this **experiment**</u>

Yes	
No	
You don't know	
DI	

	Not applicable (I already had the diagnosis)

4. Dyslipidemia / high cholesterol
Previously available information <u>latest</u>

	Yes
	No
	Doesn't know / DI

Confirmation / data collection in <u>this **follow-up**</u>

	Yes
	No
	You don't know
	DI
	I already had the diagnosis!

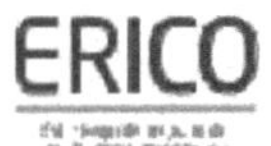

Hospital Universitário | Centro de Pesquisa Clínica
Avenida Pedroso 2565 — 3ª andar | Escola Universitária
Ararará, São Paulo, Bra. 05778-000
Fone: 55 11 3091-9375 | Fax 55 11 3083-2345

5. Smoking
Confirmation / data collection <u>in this follow-up</u>

	I Current smoker

Previously available information <u>latest</u>

	Current smoker
	Ex-labourer
	Never ran away

	Doesn't know / DI

Number of cigarettes/day

If you were an ex-smoker or never smoked, write down the date you (re)started the habit

	Former smoker

If you were a current smoker, write down the date you stopped smoking

	Never smoked
	You don't know
	DI

Participant:	
A. LEFT COMMON CAROTID ARTERY	
FIMTAVG [mm]	
FIMTMIN [mm]	
FIMTMAX [mm]	
Vessel Dia. [mm]	
Lumen Day. [mm]	

A. RIGHT COMMON CAROTID ARTERY	
FIMTAVG [mm]	

FIMTMIN [mm]	
FIMTMAX [mm]	
Vessel Dia. [mm]	
Lumen Day. [mm]	

REFERENCES

Andreas Melidonis, Ioannis A. Kyriazis, Areti Georgopali, Michalis Zairis, Anastasios Lyras, Theodoros Lambropoulos, Dimitrios Matsaidonis and Stefanos Foussas Prognostic Value of the Carotid Artery Intima-Media Thickness for the Presence and Severity of Coronary Artery Disease in Type 2 Diabetic Patients. Diabetes Care 2003; 26(11): 3189-3190).

Blaha MJ, Rivera JJ, BudoffMJ, Blankstein R, Agatston A, O'Leary DH, Cushman M, Lakoski S, Criqui MH, Szklo M, Blumenthal RS, Nasir DK. Association between obesity, high-sensitivity C-reactive protein C2 mg/L, and subclinical atherosclerosis: implications of JUPITER from the Multi Ethnic Study of Atherosclerosis. AtherosclerTreomb VascBiol. 2011; 31 :1430-1438.

Bonithon-Kopp C, Touboul P-J, Berr C et al. Relation of intima-media thickness to atherosclerotic plaques in carotid arteries The Vascular Aging (EVA) Study. Arteriosclerosis,thrombosis, andvascularbiology. 1996;16:310-316.

Bots ML, A.W. Hoes, P.J. Koudstall, A. Hofmann, D.E. Grobbee. Common carotid intima-media thickness and risk of stroke and myocardial infarction: the Rotterdam study Circulation 1997; 96: **1432-1437.**

Chambless LE, Heiss G, Folsom AR, et al. Association of coronary heart disease incidence with carotid arterial wall thickness and major risk factors: the Atherosclerosis Risk in Communities (ARIC) study, **1987-1993.** Am J Epidemiol 1997; 146:**483-94.**

Ciccone MM, Scicchitano P, Gesualdo M, Zito A, Carbonara R, Locorotondo M, et al. Serum osteoprotegerin and carotid intima media thickness in acute/chronic coronary artery diseases. J Cardiovasc Med (Hagerstown). 2013;14(1):**43-8.**

Cicorella N, Zanolla L, Franceschini L, Cacici G, De Cristan B, Arieti M, et al. Usefulness of ultrasonographic markers of carotid atherosclerosis (intima-media thickness, unstable carotid plaques and severe carotid stenosis) for predicting presence and extent of coronary artery disease. J Cardiovasc Med (Hagerstown). 2009;10(12):**906-12.**

Cutlip DE, Windecker S, Mehran R, Boam A, Cohen DJ, van Es GA, et al. Clinical end points in coronary stent trials: a case for standardized definitions. Circulation. 2007;115(17):2344-51.

Demircan S, Tekin A, Tekin G, Topcu S, Yigit F et al. Comparison of carotid intimamedia thickness in patients with stable angina pectoris versus patients with acute coronary syndrome. Am J Cardiol. 2005;96(5):**643-4.**

Den Ruijter HM, Peters SA, Anderson TJ, Britton AR, Dekker JM, Eijkemans MJ, Engstrom G, Evans GW, de Graaf J, Grobbee DE, Hedblad B, Hofman A, Holewijn S, Ikeda A, Kavousi M, Kitagawa K, Kitamura A, Koffijberg H, Lonn EM, Lorenz MW, Mathiesen EB, Nijpels G, Okazaki S, O'Leary DH, Polak JF, Price JF, Robertson C, Rembold CM, Rosvall M, Rundek T, Salonen JT, Sitzer M, Stehouwer CD, Witteman JC, Moons KG, Bots ML. Common carotid intima media thickness measurements in cardiovascular risk prediction: a meta-analysis. JAMA. 2012;308:**796-803.**

Duncan BB, Metcalf P, Crouse 3rd JR et al. Risk factors differ for carotid artery plaque with and without acoustic shadowing. Atherosclerosis Risk in Communities Study Investigators. Journal of neuroimaging: official journal of the American Society of Neuroimaging. 1997;7:28-34.

Ebrahim S, Papacosta O, Whincup P et al. Carotid plaque, intima media thickness, cardiovascular risk factors, and prevalent cardiovascular disease in men and women in the British Regional Heart Study. Stroke. 1999;30:841-850.

Feigin VL, Roth GA, Naghavi M, Parmar P, Krishnamurthi R, Chugh S, Mensah GA, Norrving B, Shiue I, Ng M, Estep K, Cercy K, Murray CJ, Forouzanfar MH; Global

Burden of Diseases, Injuries and Risk Factors Study 2013 and Stroke Experts Writing Group Global burden of stroke and risk factors in 188 countries, during 1990-2013: a systematic analysis for the Global Burden of Disease Study 2013. LancetNeurol. 2016;15(9):913-24.

Folsom AR, Kronmal RA, Detrano RC, O'Leary DH, Bild DE, Bluemke DA, Budoff MJ, Liu K, Shea S, Szklo M, Tracy RP, Watson KE, Burke GL. Coronary artery calcification compared with carotid intima- media thickness in the prediction of cardiovascular disease incidence: the Multi-Ethnic Study of Atherosclerosis (MESA). Arch InternMed. 2008;168:**1333-1339**.

Fonseca FAH, Izar MCO. Pathophysiology of acute coronary syndromes. Rev Soc Cardiol Estado de Sao Paulo 2016;26(2):74-7

G. Acoustic shadowing on B-mode ultrasound of the carotid artery predicts CHD. Ultrasound in medicine & biology. 2001;27:357-365.

Gibbons RJ, Jones DW, Gardner TJ, Goldstein LB, Moller JH, Yancy CW. The **American Heart Association's 2008 Statement of Principles for Healthcare** Reform. Circulation. 2008;118:2209-2218.

Global, regional, and national age-sex specific mortality for 264 causes of death, 19802016: a systematic analysis for the Global Burden of Disease Study 2016. Lancet 2017; 390 (10100):1151-1210.

Goff DC Jr, Bennett G, Coady S, D'Agostino RB Sr, Gibbons R, Greenland P, Lackland DT, Levy D, O'Donnell CJ, Robinson JG, Schwartz JS, Shero ST, Smith SC Jr, Sorlie P, Stone NJ, Wilson PW; American College of Cardiology/American Heart Association Task Force on Practice Guidelines .2013 ACC/AHA guideline on the assessment of cardiovascular risk: a report of the American College of Cardiology/American Heart Association Task Force on Practice Guidelines. J Am Coll Cardiol. 2014;63(25 PtB):**2935-2959**.

Goulart AC, Santos IS, Sitnik D, Staniak HL, Fedeli LG, Pastore CA, et al. Design and baseline characteristics of a coronary heart disease prospective cohort: two-year experience from the strategy of registry of acute coronary syndrome study (ERICO study) Clinics 2013;68 :**431-434**.

Greenland P, Alpert JS, Beller GA, Benjamin EJ, Budoff MJ, Fayad ZA, Foster E, Hlatky MA, Hodgson JM, Kushner FG, Lauer MS, Shaw LJ, Smith SC Jr, Taylor AJ, Weintraub WS, WengerNK, Jacobs AK, Smith SC Jr, Anderson JL, AlbertN, Buller CE, Creager MA, Ettinger SM, Guyton RA, Halperin JL, Hochman JS, Kushner FG, Nishimura R, Ohman EM, Page RL, Stevenson WG, Tarkington LG, Yancy CW; American College of Cardiology Foundation; American Heart Association .2010 ACCF/AHA guideline for assessment of cardiovascular risk in asymptomatic adults: a report of the American College of Cardiology Foundation/American Heart Association Task Force on Practice Guidelines. J Am Coll Cardiol. 2010;56:**e50-e103**.

Haberka M., Gasior Z. A carotid extra-media thickness, PATIMA combined index and coronary artery disease: comparison with well-established indexes of carotid artery and fat depots. Atherosclerosis, 243 (1) (2015), pp. 307-313

Haberka M., Lelekb M., Bochenekb B., et al. Prediction of mortality after primary percutaneous coronary intervention for acute myocardial infarction: the CADILLAC risk score. J Am Coll Cardiol. 2005;45(9):**1397-405**.

Held C , P. Hjemdahl, S.V. Eriksson, I. Bjorkander, L. Forslund, N. Rehnqvist. Prognostic implications of intima-media thickness and plaques in the carotid and femoral arteries in patients with stable angina pectoris. Eur Heart J 2001; 22 : 62 72.

Howard G. , A. Sharrett, G. Heiss, G. Evans, L. Chambless, W. Riley, et al. Carotid artery intimal-medial thickness distribution in general populations as evaluated by B-mode ultrasound Stroke 1993; 24:**1297-1304**.

Hunt KJ, Sharrett AR, Chambless LE, Folsom AR, Evans GW, Heiss In Cheol Hwang

IC, Suh SY,*, Seo AR, Ahn HY, Yim E. Association Between metabolic components and subclinical atherosclerosis in Korean Adults. Korean J Fam Med 2012;33:229-236.

Brazilian Institute of Geography and Statistics. 2010 Demographic Census, http://www.ibge.gov.br/home/estatistica/populacao/censo2010/caracteristicas_da_populacaoZresultados_do_universo.pdf. Assessed on June 10,2013.

Johnsen SH, Mathiesen EB. Carotid plaque compared with intima- media thickness as a predictor of coronary and cerebrovascular disease. Current cardiology reports. 2009;11:21-27.

Johnsen SH, Mathiesen EB. Carotid plaque compared with intima-media thickness as a predictor of coronary and cerebrovascular disease. Curr Cardiol Rep. 2009;11:21- 7.

Johnston SC, Mendis S, Mathers CD. Global variation in stroke burden and mortality: estimates from monitoring, surveillance, and modeling. Lancet Neurol. 2009; 8:345-54.

Komorovsky R, Desideri A. Carotid ultrasound assessment of patients with coronary artery disease: a useful index for risk stratification. Vasc Health Risk Manag. 2005;1(2):**131-6**.

Koskinen J, Ka'ho'nen M, Viikari JS, Taittonen L, Laitinen T, Ro'nnemaa T et al. Conventional cardiovascular risk factors and metabolic syndrome in predicting carotid intima-media thickness progression in young adults: the cardiovascular risk in young Finns study. Circulation 2009; 120: 229 -- 236.

Kuller L, Borhani N, Furberg C et al. Prevalence of subclinical atherosclerosis and cardiovascular disease and association with risk factors in the Cardiovascular Health Study. AmJ Epidemiol. 1994;139:1164-1179.

Lau KK, Chan YH, Yiu KH, Tam S, Li SW, Lau CP, Tse HF. Incremental predictive value of vascular assessments combined with the Framingham Risk Score for prediction of coronary events in subjects of low-intermediate risk. Postgrad Med J. 2008;84:**153-157**.

Longo DL, Fauci AS, Loscalzo J, Hauser SL. Harrison's Principles of Internal Medicine: Volumes 1 and 2- 18th Edition, 2012.

Lorenz MW, Markus HS, Bots ML, Rosvall M, Sitzer M. Prediction of clinical cardiovascular events with carotid intima- media thickness: a systematic review andmeta- analysis. Circulation. 2007;115:**459-467**.

Lorenz MW, Schaefer C, Steinmetz H, Sitzer M. Is carotid intima media thickness useful for individual prediction of cardiovascular risk? Ten-year results from the Carotid Atherosclerosis Progression Study (CAPS). Eur Heart J. 2010;31:2041- 2048

Lorenz MW, von Kegler S, Steinmetz H, Markus HS, Sitzer M. Carotid intima-media thickening indicates a higher vascular risk across a wide age range: prospective data from the Carotid Atherosclerosis Progression Study (CAPS). Stroke 2006;37:**87-92**.

Lotufo PA, Fernandes TG, Bando DH, Alencar AP, Bensenor IM. Income and heart disease mortality trends in Sao Paulo, Brazil, 1996 to 2010. Int J Cardiol. 2013;167:**2820-2823**.

Luepker RV, Apple FS, Christenson RH, Crow RS, Fortmann SP, Goff D, et al. Case definitions for acute coronary heart disease in epidemiology and clinical research studies: a statement from the AHA Council on Epidemiology and Prevention; AHA Statistics Committee; World Heart Federation Council on Epidemiology and Prevention; the European Society of Cardiology Working Group on Epidemiology and Prevention; Centers for Disease Control and Prevention; and the National Heart,Lung, and Blood Institute. Circulation. 2003;108 (20):2543-9.

Lusis AJ. Atherosclerosis. Nature 2000;407:**233-41**.

Mallmann AB, Fuchs SC, Gus M, Fuchs FD, Moreira LB. Population-attributable risks for ischemic stroke in a community in South Brazil: a case-control study. PLoS One. 2012;7(4):e35680.

Mancia G, Fagard R, Narkiewicz K, Redon J, Zanchetti A, Bohm M, Christiaens T, Cifkova R, De Backer G, Dominiczak A, Galderisi M, Grobbee DE, Jaarsma T,

Kirchhof P, Kjeldsen SE, Laurent S, Manolis AJ, Nilsson PM, Ruilope LM, Schmieder RE, Sirnes PA, Sleight P, Viigimaa M, Waeber B, Zannad F; Task Force for the Management of Arterial Hypertension of the European Society of Hypertension and the European Society of Cardiology .2013 ESHESC practice guidelines for the management of arterial hypertension. Blood Press. 2014;23:**3- 16**.

Mancini GB, Dahlof B, Diez J. Surrogate markers for cardiovascular disease: structural markers. Circulation 2004; 109(25 Suppl 1):IV22-30.

Ministry of Health. Executive Secretariat. Datasus. Health Information. Morbidity and information. Available at:
http://bvsms.saude.gov.br/bvs/publicacoes/saude_brasil_2013_analise_situacao_s aude.pdf. Assessed on July 27 2016.

Morrow DA, Antman EM, Charlesworth A, Cairns R, Murphy SA, de Lemos JA, et al. TIMI risk score for ST-elevation myocardial infarction: A convenient, bedside, clinical score for risk assessment at presentation: An intravenous nPA for treatment of infarcting myocardium early II trial substudy. Circulation. 2000;102(17):2031-7.

Naqvi TZ, Lee MS. Carotid intima-media thickness and plaque in cardiovascular risk assessment. JACC Cardiovasc Imaging. 2014;7:**1025-1038**.

O'Leary DH, Bots ML. Imaging of atherosclerosis: carotid intima-media thickness. Eur HeartJ. 2010;31:1682-1689.

O'Donnell MJ, Chin SL, Rangarajan S, Xavier D, Liu L, Zhang H, Rao-Melacini P, Zhang X, Pais P, Agapay S, Lopez-Jaramillo P,Damasceno A, Langhorne P, McQueen MJ, Rosengren A, Dehghan M, Hankey GJ, Dans AL, Elsayed A, Avezum A, Mondo C, Diener HC, Ryglewicz D, Czlonkowska A, Pogosova N, Weimar C, Iqbal R, Diaz R, Yusoff K, Yusufali A, Oguz A, Wang X, Penaherrera E, Lanas F, Ogah OS, Ogunniyi A, Iversen HK,Malaga G, Rumboldt Z, Oveisgharan S, Al Hussain F, Magazi D, Nilanont Y, Ferguson J, Pare G, Yusuf; INTERSTROKE investigators. Global and regional effects of potentially modifiable risk factors associated with acute stroke in 32 countries (INTERSTROKE): a case-control study. Lancet. 2016;388 (10046):761-75.

O'Leary DH, Polak JF, Kronmal RA, et al. Thickening of the carotid wall. A marker for atherosclerosis in the elderly? Cardiovascular Health Study Collaborative Research Group. Stroke 1996;27(2):**224-31**.

O'Leary DH, Polak JF, Kronmal RA, Kittner SJ, Bond MG, Wolfson SK Jr, Bommer W, Price TR, Gardin JM, Savage PJ. Distribution and correlates of sonographically detected carotid artery disease in the Cardiovascular Health Study. The CHS Collaborative Research Group. Stroke. 1992;23:**1752-1760**.

Oliveira, I.R.S.; Meireles, D.P; Silva, C.F.M; Souza, A.M.; Manual do Protocolo de Ultrassonografia de Carótidas - Espessura da Camada Média-ntima, HU-USP Reading Center (Estudo Longitudinal da Saúde do Adulto - ELSA), 2008.

Park HW, Kim WH, Kim KH, Yang DJ, Kim JH, Song IG, et al. Carotid plaque is associated with increased cardiac mortality in patients with coronary artery disease. IntJ Cardiol. 2013;166(3):**658-63**.

Peters SAE, den Ruijter HN, Bots ML and Moons KGM. Improvements in risk stratification for the occurrence of cardiovascular disease by imaging subclinical atherosclerosis: a systematic review Heart 2012; 98: 177-184.

Pignoli P, Tremoli E, Poli A, Oreste P, Paoletti R. Intimal plus medial thickness of the arterial wall: a direct measurement with ultrasound imaging. Circulation. 1986;74:1399-1406.

Polak JF, M.J. Pencina, K.M. Pencina, C.J. O'Donnell, P.A. Wolf, R.B. D'Agostino Sr. Carotid-wall intima-media thickness and cardiovascular events. Engl J Med 2011; 365: **213-221**.

Ribeiro AL, Duncan BB, Brant LC, Lotufo PA, Mill JG, Barreto SM. Cardiovascular Health in Brazil: Trends and Perspectives. Circulation. 2016;133(4):422-33.

Robertson W.B. The International Atherosclerosis Project. Pathologia et Microbiologia 1967;30:**810-816**.

Rosa EM, Kramer C, Castro I. Association between coronary artery atherosclerosis and the intima-media thickness of the common carotid artery measured on ultrasonography. Arq Bras Cardiol. 2003;80(6):**589-92**.

Rosvall M, Janzon L, Berglund G, Engstrom G, Hedblad B. Incident coronary events and case fatality in relation to common carotid intima- media thickness. J Intern Med. 2005;257:**430-437**.

S. Pursnani, M. Diener-West, A.R. Sharrett The effect of aging on the association between coronary heart disease risk factors and carotid intima media thickness: an analysis of the atherosclerosis risk in communities (ARIC) cohort. Atherosclerosis, 2014; 233: **441-446**.

Salonen JT, Salonen R. Ultrasonographically assessed carotid morphology and the risk of coronary heart disease. Arterioscler Thromb. 1991;11:1245-1249

Santos. IS, Goulart AC, Brandao RM, Santos RCO, Bittencourt MS, Sitnik D, Pereira AC, Pastore CA, Samesima N, Lotufo PA, Bensenor IM. One-year Mortality after an Acute Coronary Event and its Clinical Predictors: The ERICO Study. Arq Bras Cardiol. 2015; 105(1):53-64.

Shah PK. Screening asymptomatic subjects for subclinical atherosclerosis: can we, does it matter, and should we? Journal of the American College of Cardiology. 2010;56:98-105.

Simon A, Megnien JL, Chironi G. The value of carotid intima- media thickness for predicting cardiovascular risk. Arterioscler Thromb Vasc Biol. 2010;30:**182-185**.

Smith SC, Jr, Greenland P, Grundy SM. AHA Conference Proceedings. Prevention conference V: Beyond secondary prevention: Identifying the high-risk patient for primary prevention: executive summary. American Heart Association. Circulation. 2000;101(1):111-6.

Stein JH, Korcarz CE, Hurst RT, Lonn E, Kendall CB, Mohler ER, Najjar SS, Rembold CM, Post WS. Use of carotid ultrasound to identify subclinical vascular disease and evaluate cardiovascular disease risk: a consensus statement from the American Society of Echocardiography Carotid Intima-Media Thickness Task Force. J Am Soc Echocardiogr. 2008; 21:**93-111**.

Tello-Montoliu A, Molto JM, Lopez-Hernandez N, Garcia-Medina A, Roldan V, Sogorb F, Lip GY, Marin F. Common carotid artery intima-media thickness and intracranial pulsatility index in non-ST-elevation acute coronary syndromes. Cerebrovasc Dis. 2007;24 (4):338-42.

Thygesen K, Alpert JS, White HD. Universal definition of myocardial infarction. Eur HeartJ. 2007;28(20):2525-38.

Toth PP. Subclinical atherosclerosis: what it is, what it means and what we can do about it. Int J Clin Pract 2008;62:**1246-54**.

Touboul PJ, M.G. Hennerici, S. Meairs, H. Adams, P. Amarenco, N. Bornstein, et al. Mannheim carotid intima-media thickness and plaque consensus (2004-20062011). An update on behalf of the advisory board of the 3rd, 4th and 5th watching the risk symposia, at the 13th, 15th and 20th European Stroke Conferences, Mannheim, Germany, 2004, Brussels, Belgium, 2006, and Hamburg, Germany, 2011 CerebrovascDis2012;34 : **290-296**.

Touboul PJ, M.G. Hennerici, S. Meairs, H. Adams, P. Amarenco, N. Bornstein, et al. Mannheim carotid intima-media thickness consensus (**2004-2006**) Cerebrovasc Dis2007; 23: **75-80**.

Trichopoulou A, Costacou T, Bamia C, Trichopopoulos D. Adherence to a Mediterranean diet and survival in a Greek population. N Engl J Med. 2003; 348: 2599-608.

Vos T,Barber RM, Bell B, Bertozzi-Villa A, Biryukov S, Bolliger I, et al. Global, regional, and national incidence, prevalence, and years lived with disability for 301 acute and chronic diseases and injuries in 188 countries, 1990-2013: a systematic analysis for the Global Burden of Disease Study 2013. Lancet 2015;386:**743-800**.

Wang Y, Beydoun MA. The obesity epidemic in the United Statesgender, age, socioeconomic, racial/ethnic, and geographic characteristics: a systematic review and meta-regression analysis. Epidemiol Rev 2007;29:6e28.

Welsh RC, Goldstein P, Carvalho AC. Impact on Clinical Outcomes of Randomization at Community Hospitals Versus Pre-hospital location in STEMI Patients: Insights from the STREAM Study. Circulation. 2015;132(suppl 3): A13594.

WHO, 2010. International Statistical Classification of Diseases and Related Health Problems. 10thRevision.

Willett WC, Sacks F, Trichopoulou A, Drescher G, Ferro-Luzzi A, Helsing E, et al.Mediterranean diet pyramid:a cultural model for helthy eating.Am J Clin Nutr. 1995; 6: 1402S-6S.

World Health Organization- Cardiovascular Diseases. -Health systems: improving performance. Geneva: WHO, 2005.

World Health Organization (WHO). The top 10 causes of death. Fact sheet №310. Available at: http://www.who.int/mediacentre/factsheets/fs310/en/ . Assessed on April 10, 2016.

World Health Organization. World Heart Federation World Stroke Organization. Global atlas on cardiovascular disease prevention and control: policies, strategies, and interventions. Published 2011. Availableat: http://www.who.int/cardiovascular_diseases/publications/atlas_cvd/en/. Assessed on April 10, 2016.

Xu L, Jiang CQ, Lam TH, Lin JM, Yue XJ, Cheng KK, Liu B,Jin YL, Zhang WS, Thomas GN. The Metabolic syndrome is associated with subclinical atherosclerosis independent of insulin resistance: the Guangzhou Biobank Cohort Study-CVD. Clinical Endocrinology 2010; 73: **181-188**.

Yan AT, Yan RT, Tan M, Eagle KA, Granger CB, Dabbous OH, et al. In-hospital revascularization and one-year outcome of acute coronary syndrome patients stratified by the GRACE risk score. Am J Cardiol. 2005;96(7):**913-6**.

Yeboah J, McClelland RL, PPolonsky TS, Burke GL, Sibley CT, O'Leary D, Carr JJ, Goff DC, Greenland P, Herrington DM. Comparison of novel risk markers for improvement in cardiovascular risk assessment in intermediate- risk individuals. JAMA. 2012;308:**788-795**.

Yuk HB, Park HW, Jung IJ, et al. Analysis of carotid ultrasound findings on cardiovascular events in patients with coronary artery disease during seven year follow-up. Korean Circ J.2015.

Yusuf S, Rangarajan S, Teo K. Cardiovascular risk and events in 17 low-middle-and-income countries. N Engl J Med 2014; 371:818-27.

APPENDICES

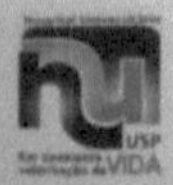

São Paulo, 23 de junho de 2016.

Il$^{mo(a)}$. S$^{r(a)}$.
Dra. Alessandra Carvalho Goulart
Divisão de Clinica Médica do Hospital Universitário
UNIVERSIDADE DE SÃO PAULO

REFERENTE: Projeto de Pesquisa "Valor prognóstico da espessura da camada íntima média das paredes carotídeas em indivíduos pós síndrome coronariana aguda no Estudo 'Estratégia de registro de insuficiência coronariana (ERICO)': avaliação de risco em um ano de seguimento"
Pesquisador(a) responsável: Alessandra Carvalho Goulart
Pesquisador executante: Danilo Peron Meireles
CAAE: 56883116.7.0000.0076
Registro CEP-HU/USP: 156516

Prezado(a) Senhor(a)

O Comitê de Ética em Pesquisa do Hospital Universitário da Universidade de São Paulo, em reunião ordinária realizada no dia 17 de junho de 2016 analisou o Projeto de Pesquisa acima citado, considerando-o como **APROVADO**.

Lembramos que cabe ao pesquisador elaborar e apresentar a este Comitê, relatórios parciais e final, de acordo com a Resolução nº 466/2012 do Conselho Nacional de Saúde, inciso XI.2, letra "d".

O primeiro relatório está previsto para 17 de dezembro de 2016.

Atenciosamente,

Dr. Mauricio Seckler
Coordenador do Comitê de Ética em Pesquisa
Hospital Universitário da USP

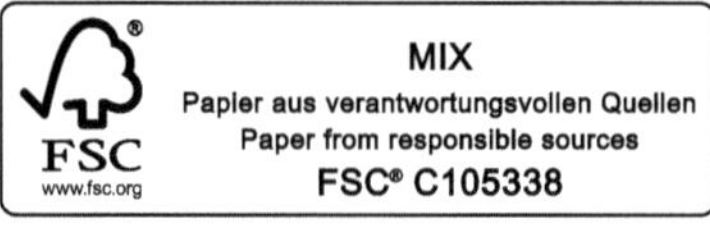

Printed by Books on Demand GmbH, Norderstedt / Germany